THE
SECRET
ART OF
SHIATSU

SEI-KI

Life in Resonance

KISHI

AND

ϽΟΝ

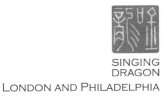

SINGING
DRAGON
LONDON AND PHILADELPHIA

First published in 2011
by Singing Dragon
an imprint of Jessica Kingsley Publishers
116 Pentonville Road
London N1 9JB, UK
and
400 Market Street, Suite 400
Philadelphia, PA 19106, USA

www.singingdragon.com

Library of Congress Cataloging in Publication Data
Kishi, Akinobu.
  Sei-ki : life in resonance, the secret art of shiatsu / Akinobu Kishi and Alice Whieldon.
    p. cm.
  Includes bibliographical references and index.
  ISBN 978-1-84819-042-9 (alk. paper)
  1. Acupressure. I. Whieldon, Alice. II. Title.
  RM723.A27K57 2011
  615.8'222--dc22

                                  2011008130

British Library Cataloguing in Publication Data
A CIP catalogue record for this book is available from the British Library

ISBN 978 1 84819 042 9

Printed and bound in Great Britain

CONTENTS

Introduction 5

PART I HISTORIES 9
    Manual Therapy in Japan to the Twentieth Century 10
    The Emergence of Shiatsu in Twentieth-Century Japan .. 23
    Post-War Shiatsu 27
    Tokujiro Namikoshi (1905–2000) 33
    Shizuto Masunaga (1925–1981) 36
    Akinobu Kishi (born 1949) 46

PART II IN CONVERSATION 57
    Shiatsu 59
    Breathing Again: Seiki-Soho 88

PART III MUNICH WORKSHOP: JULY 2010 119

PART IV MEETING KISHI 145
    Accounts of Seiki-Soho 146

POSTSCRIPT BY AKINOBU KISHI 160
GLOSSARY 161
APPENDIX I FLOWCHART OF THE HISTORY OF TRADITIONAL
    JAPANESE FOLK MEDICINE 165
APPENDIX II DR TARO TAKEMI'S ARTICLE ON THE
    NEED FOR KANPO 167
ACKNOWLEDGEMENTS 170
INDEX 171

Introduction

In the summer of 2008, I attended a workshop with Kishi *sensei*[1] in Brighton, UK. I had been to many such gatherings over the previous ten years. In that time I had written a few articles and started, but stalled on, a book about *Seiki*,[2] his style of *Shiatsu*. It was all familiar territory and I sat, relaxed, with 30 or so other participants in a circle around the room as Kishi invited and addressed comments and queries. After one question, I forget the specifics, he paused, perhaps a little weary at the thought of translating tricky ideas into his third language. Then he waved in my general direction and said, 'Alice will write an article on that.'

'No,' I said, suddenly alert and prompted into recalcitrance not only by a feeling that the effort that went into one article was out of proportion to the number of people who would actually read it, but also by a sudden conviction: 'No one reads articles.' I rashly announced, 'We should write a book.'

Kishi looked at me and smiled, maybe a little surprised, then nodded, 'OK! A book then,' he replied. And so it began.

I came across Shiatsu at the age of 18, through a treatment I was given while cooking for a Pauline Sasaki[3] workshop in 1985. I knew

---

1 Sensei means teacher in Japanese.
2 Seiki, or Sei-ki, is the core subject of this book. It is the name that Akinobu Kishi has given to his own work which came out of his research into Shiatsu. The *kanji*, or Japanese lettering, for this word can be written in many ways, and Kishi has developed his own kanji for it. It is difficult to translate, roughly meaning *regulating ki*, but regulation here means returning to one's original movement, brightening your life and regaining your aliveness. It is a return to your natural consciousness: the topic of this book.
3 Pauline Sasaki (1946–2010) was a Shiatsu teacher based in New York who had a significant influence on Shiatsu in Europe. She worked extensively with Wataru Ohashi and also with Kishi and Shizuto Masunaga. She and Clifford Andrews are the originators of Quantum Shiatsu.

nothing about it, accepting the offer only because it seemed churlish not to, but was astonished at how it touched and spoke to me in a way I had never experienced before. Looking back now I wonder why I did not simply find a practitioner and get some sessions; it would have been a cheaper, easier option, but I was determined to study it, and a few years later enrolled in the practitioners' training then offered by the Shiatsu College, London.

I enjoyed my three years' training and built a practice while continuing my Shiatsu studies with postgraduate work. But it was never quite what I had hoped it would be; I never quite regained the moment of connection experienced in that very first session. After a few years I was tired and bored, ready to move on and in the process of stepping into a completely different career, when the whisperings about Kishi that I had been dismissing for nearly a decade finally became too interesting to ignore. In fact I was warned off him – he was said to be a dangerous maverick – but that only fuelled my curiosity and, shortly thereafter, the opportunity presented itself to meet him and receive a session.

The moment I lay down and he sat beside me, before he even laid his hands on me, I knew I was home. I breathed a sigh of relief as I recognised the spark I had always been looking for, and I have not looked back.

———

Kishi has forged his own way for 30 years, from the point at which he began to call his work, *Seiki*. For him and for many who followed him, this beginning drew a permanent line under Shiatsu and it did not seem necessary to refer to the past. But the process of looking at a life and an approach reveals patterns you do not necessarily expect and, in writing this book, Shiatsu came to the fore in sharp relief, both as a vital constituent of Kishi's development and as the context in which his work sits.

Kishi has never, in fact, been the out and out foreigner to his background that his rejection of Shiatsu and embrace of European culture may have suggested. Although Seiki began with a break away from Shiatsu, it rose directly out of years of his close investigation of it. Ever keen to engage with the broader aesthetic that Shiatsu shares with other Japanese arts, he has always loved the tea ceremony, offered sake to the *kami*[4] at Shinto shrines, and enjoyed any number of other traditional practices and pleasures, from pork dumplings to a well-made kimono. Kishi's beautifully camouflaged genius has been in cultivating common humanity through the prism and clarity of his own discipline and desires. Our connections with each other are what we want and pursue regardless of cultural boundaries. Whether wearing a kimono or a kilt, this connective possibility is simply human.

Kishi's relationship with Shiatsu has been ambiguous though, and sometimes mutually antagonistic. He is a dissident but, as history demonstrates, dissenters are those who know and love their traditions well enough to depart from them in order to remain faithful. It was never the heart of Shiatsu he left behind. He has pursued that and *Seiki-Soho* is the result. Somewhat paradoxically, this has brought him full circle to join the teachers he once stepped away from, now finding his place among them as a key actor in the history of Shiatsu.

Alice Whieldon
Ontario, Canada
July 2010

---

4   The kami are the Shinto gods and goddesses or ancestors.

There is only one thing that I know
I came through these 30 years with this one thing
I recognise a choked feeling of energy stagnation and a missing
    place; I feel it and fill it.
The breath becomes one
I touch space
I concentrate
The body begins to move
Thus it is over
It is good enough
And many people's words were, *I'm breathing again*
It has been my life and my joy.

Akinobu Kishi
Maebashi, Japan
January 2010

PART I

HISTORIES

Manual Therapy in Japan to the Twentieth Century

As the first and most direct response to discomfort, manual therapy reaches into the prehistory of all races and nations. Human contact is the foundation of medicine; its simplest expression and, in the right hands, the most profound appreciation of what it is to be whole. In Japan, Shiatsu is one of the more recent ways in which the human impulse to touch for health has found form.

The elements that came together to describe it can be traced back through the history of Eastern medicine in Japan, folk medicine and through the principles that govern the Japanese arts where art, philosophy, medicine and the principles of Western science intersect.

Before the sixth century CE arrival of Buddhist monks from China, Japanese history is hard to pin down since little was recorded by the people themselves. Such material as there is must be interpreted from archaeological evidence, a few Chinese texts and Japanese mythology.[5]

The earliest known reference to manual therapy comes from this last source and predates Chinese influence. In the 720 CE compilation of earlier mythology, *Nihon Shoki*, or the *Chronicles of Japan*, an ancient poem[6] is recorded in which the medicine 'ancestor', Sukunahikona no Mikoto, is described as healing directly through manual touch. Some

---

5   Morton, S.W. and Olenik, K.J. (2005) *Japan: Its History and Culture.* New York: McGraw-Hill, p.6.

6   The ancient poem is: Sukunahikona no nigatenite nadereba ochiru dokunomushi osebanakunaru yamai no chisio oriyo sagareyo idehayaku.

Shiatsu therapists point to this as the expository myth of their art, placing it at the heart of Japanese culture and spirit.

While the influence of Korea on the development of Japan's culture is significant and preceded that of China, the latter had a deeper and more lasting effect on medicine. When Chinese travellers arrived, they brought with them a sophisticated culture, religion and system of medicine that wrought deep and permanent changes on their willing, but less sophisticated, cousins. Physic, while disseminated to a large degree through personal contact, was also recorded in detailed books of diagnosis and treatment that had been honed over centuries and facilitated study. So widely circulated were they that many early texts survive to this day.

Chinese medicine,[7] however, while complex, was not a fixed system and texts were references rather than authorities in themselves. The system was a medical response to a world in flux. Its many diagnostic tools and techniques for treatment spoke to the correspondingly multifarious needs of its people in the disparate climes and circumstances of China's vast territories. Its core resources were *Moxibustion*,[8] *Acupuncture*,[9] herbs,[10] and manual therapy which, when combined with the wisdom and skill of the doctor in perceiving the myriad subtleties of situation and character, offered a practical, holistic approach to health. Texts, while serving to remind and elucidate, did not automatically supersede this nuanced understanding.

In response to Chinese influence, from the seventh century CE,[11] Japanese scholars travelled to China to study at the source. Many of them did so in government sponsored missions, building on knowledge in all areas to contribute to the developing governance and culture of their nation. So impressed were they by the detailed

---

7   Chinese medicine referred to here is not the traditional Chinese medicine (TCM) that practitioners in the West, and today in China, know. TCM was formalised in the 1950s by the communist regime with a nationalistic agenda.

8   Moxibustion refers to the burning of herbs on or near *tsubos* (usually translated as 'points').

9   The use of needles on points on the body for medical purposes.

10 Herbal medicine is now referred to as *Kanpo*, although the word Kanpo originally referred to the Japanese version of all Chinese medicine.

11 During the seventh and eighth centuries, the Japanese government sent many missions to China to study cultural and governmental affairs (Zui and Tou periods).

diagnostics and treatments of Chinese medicine that, as early as the Nara period (710–784 CE), it was adopted as the official medical system in Japan and instituted into law books by which medical education was conducted. But, even up to the eighteenth century, this 'official' medicine was practised by only a small number of professional doctors and reserved for the wealthy and ruling classes. The majority of people had no access to medical assistance and little choice but to rely on folk medicine; less sophisticated, standardised or expensive than Chinese medicine and practised mostly by monks.

While contact with China continued to enhance understanding, by 894, when the government sponsored missions stopped, Japanese culture was developing its own distinct character and methodologies. In Japanese hands, Chinese philosophy and practices were imbued with an essentially local flavour. So, from this point, Chinese medicine in Japan must be seen increasingly through the filter of Japanese interpretation and use. The self-imposed isolation of Japan between around 1633 and 1853, from all but a few controlled contacts with the outside world, also served to strengthen indigenous themes and approaches in all areas.

A form of manual therapy, which the Chinese brought with them as *Doin-Ankyo*, came first from India and developed in Central China before travelling to Japan. Developing a Japanese slant it became known as *Anma-Doin*,[12] and the oldest Japanese medical book still in existence, Tamba Yasuyori's *Ishin-ho* of 982 CE, states that this stands equal to the other medical methods in principle. At roughly this point, manual therapy was incorporated into traditional Japanese medicine as *Koho* (classical) *Anma*.

Manual therapy formed an important aspect of medieval Japanese medicine but there was an early tendency to sideline it as an adjunct to the more technical methods. Although one of the main diagnostic tools, it was impossible to define by technique alone since it was not limited to physical palpation. This difficulty in defining it conversely made it easier to underplay. But, in a system in which diagnosis and treatment cannot properly be considered as separate, manual therapy

---

12 Doin refers to a system of exercise or movement for health such as yoga or *Seitai Soho* (see p.132 for further explanation).

按腹導引の内

「利関術」の（1）

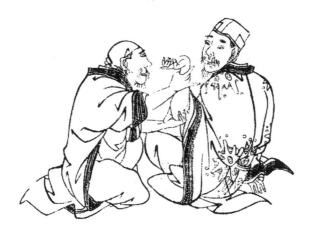

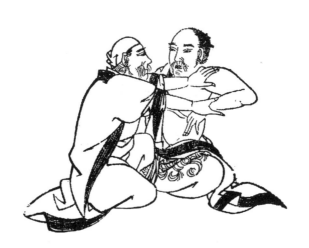

「利関術」の（2）

井沢正著「按腹図解と指圧療法」より

Anpuku-Doin (Rikan no Jyutsu) from *Anpuku-Zukai* by Fusai Ota was an indispensable element. Even so, as early as the eighth century, there is evidence that Koho Anma was being awarded a lower status than herbs, Acupuncture and Moxibustion, reflected in the curtailment of the length of training required for it, which was now less than for the other medical arts. The reason for this is not certain, but probably mirrored changes in China whose influence remained strong, at least until the seventeenth century, and where the technical forms of medicine were increasingly elevated at the expense of manual therapy.

While texts were perhaps not originally meant to usurp the authority of the doctor, the reality was that the written word was a presage of the modern world and served an increasingly important role in training. It is tempting to hark back to golden ages, such as a time when medicine was sagely passed on in careful transmission, but the problems of handing skills on to a new generation have exercised frustrated teachers in all times and cultures. Since manual therapy was not extensively recorded, having no tools and relying on the subjective skill of the practitioner, it did not lend itself to wide dissemination as a formal art and suffered in consequence; indeed, little is known about the development of Koho Anma in the period between the tenth and seventeenth centuries.

It has also been suggested that, by the time books were being produced for the teaching of medicine, the medical arts were already being affected by the hazards of widespread dissemination.[13] The result was a limiting of what was written down to that which was safe and more or less visible. Medicine in relatively unskilled hands, which book learning promotes, could not, either conscionably or practically, include the subtleties known by the great physicians and texts were effectively dumbed down versions of the medical arts.

While change may have been fairly slow before, what is certain is that the Edo period (1603–1868), the era of the Tokugawa Shogunate, brought with it a distinct change in tone. Where the native religious consciousness, *Shinto*, eschews text to the point of regarding the written word with suspicion, while valuing the hidden or even

---

13 Endo, R. (2008) *Tao Shiatsu: Revolution in Oriental Medicine.* Available at www.taoshiatsu. com/wp-content/uploads/downloads/2010/12/taoshiatsu_revolution.pdf, accessed on 7 June 2011.

secret, the new regime deliberately rejected secrecy as politically suspect in favour of a more Confucian model of structured hierarchies in which transparency was equated with virtue. With the imposition of organised peace in Japan, after years of internal strife, also came an emphasis on formal learning in which the written word was a vital feature. This was a shift much aided by the introduction from Europe of the printing press and the possibility, for the first time, of producing and distributing information on a large scale. Edo period changes, however, were distillations of tendencies that had their roots in earlier times. For instance, as early as the thirteenth century, Shinto had begun to bow to pressure to formalise itself in text,[14] largely in response to the growth of text-rich Buddhism.

Although this regime has sometimes been characterised as blandly rigid, it has equally been applauded as fostering a flowering of Japanese culture. In this new order, old power structures that centred on charismatic leaders, subjective judgement and transmission in close apprenticeships were perceived as a threat to the values and power structures of the new epoch. Koho Anma, with its lack of standing as an academic subject, no tools or fixed technique, was difficult to standardise and reflected the old world of subjective authority. As values changed, its gradual slide from high standing carried a certain inevitability.

Despite the slow loss of authority down the centuries, manual therapy nonetheless continued to develop. Used not only by manual specialists, but also by all medical practitioners, the area of greatest skill within it was *hara* treatment, known as *Anpuku* or *Haratori*, developed as early as the tenth century (Heian period).

Usually translated as the abdominal area, hara is a much fuller concept and reality than this anatomical definition could suggest, for it sits at the heart of Japanese sensibility, culture and identity. The challenge of translating it into a Western context exposes differences in the ways in which East and West have made sense of the world at such a deep sub-strata of meaning creation, representing such basic assumptions on both sides, that they can be hard to explain.

---

14   In Bowning, R. (2008) *The Religious Traditions of Japan 500–1600.* Cambridge: Cambridge University Press.

Hara is as essential and ordinary to traditional Japan as it can be obscure and extraordinary to foreign students of that culture. In its most basic use in the West, it is understood as the centre of gravity which the martial artist or Shiatsu therapist learns to use to good effect in body mechanics. But this definition barely scratches the surface of its expression in Japan where hara is the centre of mind/spirit/body that defines humanity.

To be in your hara is to be in right relationship with yourself and with the world, evidence of which is manifested in every thought, word and action of daily life. To live in hara culture, is to live with integrity. But such a definition does little justice to what is experiential and denotes a *right feeling* that is inseparable from correct performance and rendered peculiar by attempts to describe and analyse it.

As part of its location as the core of being, showing the anatomical hara to a doctor in Japan, with its attendant implications, is a demonstration of enormous mutual trust. More so as it is regarded as a matter of honourable conduct to keep personal concerns private. Consequently, the relationship between doctor and patient was at the heart of traditional diagnosis and allowed the trusted medic to understand the patient in all their nuanced complexity.[15] So manual therapy that included Anpuku was medicine of the highest order. It went directly to the core of imbalance, demanding an intimate and respectful understanding of the individual, combined with skill in touch, in order to restore harmony in the most fundamental sense.

Japanese governments have always understood the power of medicine and, over the centuries, have done their best to control it. Restrictions introduced during the Edo period reserved Koho Anma as a profession for blind people and, at the same time, forbade all but the highest level of master practitioner, the *kengyou*, to practise Anpuku.

---

15   It is of interest to note that some European doctors in the same period laid similar stress on the importance of knowing the patient as an individual and the pointlessness of medicine without this. The early modern period in Europe was one in which the move to a scientific model was by no means ubiquitous or seamless and medicine remained, for a long time, a mix of superstition, magic, religion and the new science with any number of different practitioners from wise women and low-level surgeons to university taught medics. All were consulted according to need and preference (regardless of social class except where cost dictated necessity) rather than consensus as to which might be more respectable or mainstream.

The kengyou were powerful dictators in their field, governing the personal and professional lives of those who relied on their patronage for a living. Yet, in an important shift, these practitioners did not work in medicine, but as skilled and exclusive dispensers of comfort and sensual pleasure to the wealthy. Also, since few qualified as kengyou, Koho Anma slipped further in prestige since the removal of Anpuku from manual treatments rendered these less effective. By the nineteenth century, the art of diagnosis in what was now just called *Anma*, was largely gone and with it, the profession's standing as medicine. Although a few practitioners kept Koho Anma alive in family traditions, moves to return it to its former status were unsuccessful.

Had Koho Anma been permitted to develop without restrictions, there probably would have been no need for Shiatsu to emerge as a specific therapy. But, while the erosion of its authority raises interesting questions, modern Shiatsu developed, not out of the much reduced Anma, but in a more fragmented lineage from the diagnostics of Koho Anma and specialised touch of Anpuku, combined with other influences drawn by innovative twentieth-century practitioners from Eastern philosophy, traditional methods of self-healing and Western anatomy and physiology.

The influence of Western medicine in Japan began with the first visitors from early modern Europe;[16] mostly Portuguese in the sixteenth century followed by Dutch traders from the seventeenth to nineteenth centuries. But the impact of the medicine they brought with them was limited until the mid-nineteenth century. In the early days, Portuguese missionaries did have some influence; most were trained in the medical arts and, since the majority of ordinary Japanese suffered the usual ills of poverty, exacerbated by years of internal warfare, and rarely had access to formal medical help, they were happy to accept the assistance offered in missionary clinics. But this did not last and, when Christianity was banned and violently suppressed in the early seventeenth century, contact with the West was reduced almost exclusively to those permitted to trade from the artificial island of

---

16   The early modern period in Europe refers to the period after the Middle Ages, from about 1500 to 1800.

Dejima, off Nagasaki, and the minor influence that Western medicine had gained was largely lost.

Dutch traders took Dejima over from the Portuguese in the mid-seventeenth century and were permitted to bring their own doctors with them. Reflecting the hesitant steps of early science, these medics were heavily reliant on the ancient theories of the four humours and on rudimentary anatomy influenced, and also hampered, by the limited understanding of second-century CE Greek physician, Galen.[17] While these men were rarely allowed to set foot on the Japanese mainland, the medicine they practised was of some interest to their Japanese translators and a few shogunate officials.

During the more than 200 years of Japanese isolation, although these Dejima medics made a scarcely detectable impact on the wider Japanese consciousness, they gained an influence out of proportion to their numbers, and probably to their knowledge, with the few Japanese with whom they had regular contact. Many of the translators who worked with them became their students. In some cases, entire schools of medicine were established on the say-so of a few men and this limited wisdom was passed down orally as family heritage. Their occasional trips to the capital, Edo, were also occasions when scholars could glean as much as they could from these exotic foreigners and, in true Japanese style, as much as possible was squeezed out of such men and eagerly disseminated without, apparently, much thought that these might be very partial and flawed versions of the medicine of their homelands. The formal teaching that went on was on a one-to-one basis since translations were made only slowly, but anatomical drawings were of great interest as they were radically different from Chinese charts and a great deal more accurate.

Although it seems that, to one degree or another, these visiting Western medics allied themselves to the 'newer' medical models of the infant sciences, it is worth noting that European medicine at this time was still a long way from anything that would be recognised today. Most Europeans of this period, looking for medical intervention, drew on whatever mix of magic, religion and science that the situation

---

17   Galen (130–200 CE) was a Greek physician who wrote numerous books on medicine and provided the foundation for early Islamic and early modern Western medicine.

seemed to demand. It was not so different, in the nature of being a cocktail of the more sensible with the wildly superstitious, from the Japanese approach. Nonetheless, the Western medical arts were slowly being formalised and universalised, based on dissection, vivisection and the categorisation of disease. Medics had begun to quiz the human form, not as an integrated whole, but as a dissectible machine, focusing on the emphatically material mechanics of flesh and bone. As such they aimed to demystify the body and offer interventions that, though they saved lives, universalised medicine away from the particularities of an individual's condition to an ideological view of diseases as discrete characters and events in themselves. Overarching theories are so much easier to teach, research and apply than the messier realities of an actual human being. But such meta-narratives rarely rule without comment, especially in the questioning crucible of the Western mind.

Though Western influence was limited to just a few Japanese during the years of isolation, those who did study its medicine were impressed by the anatomical approach and its demonstrable accuracy, but the philosophical and cultural differences were vast. For example, in China and Japan, practical use and *ki* were emphasised in charts of the human body rather than visual accuracy. So Western medicine was vulnerable to misappropriation and was shaped by this new context.

Many books of Western medicine were eventually translated during the eighteenth and nineteenth centuries,[18] but the general populace had no contact with it after the expulsion of the Jesuits,[19] and it was a fringe interest. It was only in the nineteenth century that it was taken up on an official level as the injunctions against foreigners were relaxed. Attempts by official Kanpo[20] doctors to suppress scientific medicine were unsuccessful, since, on the level of muscle and bone at least, the scientific model was more accurate than the charts and hypotheses of Chinese medicine and based on a fundamentally different ideology of

---

18 One of the most important results of the drive to translate was the 1774 publication of *Kaitai Shinsho* (*A New Treatise on Anatomy*). Between 1774 and the end of the Meiji era, 47 different kinds of Western medical works were translated into Japanese.

19 The Jesuits (founded in 1540), or the Society of Jesus, are a Roman Catholic group basing their work on the teachings of their founder, Ignatius of Loyola.

20 Kanpo is the name given to the Japanese version of Chinese medicine.

life that was in line with the technological revolution that Japan was quick to embrace.

After Japan opened again to foreigners, the new Meiji government demonstrated its confidence in Western medicine as the preferred model, based on German practice of the time, and Japanese scientists and medics threw themselves into research to bring them up to a comparable level. The scientific view of health and disease became the underpinning of all medicine, including medical approaches.

Western massage was introduced to Japan by the French during the Meiji period (1868–1912). As a manual therapy, it was similar enough to what Anma had become to be easily assimilated and they were differentiated from each other more through the venues in which they were performed than by wide variations in technique. 'Massage' was increasingly the name given to therapy performed in a sports context for its suggestion of a 'modern' approach, while Anma was the term retained in the provinces and at traditional hot springs.

Manual therapy also existed in the higher echelons of Japanese society as *Teate*, closer to spiritual healing than medicine. The Emperor's touch was said to bring healing and pointed to a belief that touch represented more immediate and powerful healing than the medical approach.

Anpuku survived in a small way, privately handed down in families, although evidence is patchy. The first figure who can be pointed to as having a hand in its public promotion and revival is Kanpo doctor, Todo Yoshimasu (1702–1773). His influential writings on herbal medicine advocated hara diagnosis through touch or *Fuku-Shin*. In asserting that all illnesses could be addressed through the hara as the source of vitality, his is the first record pointing to hara work as a specifically Japanese medical approach. The timing of his publication is also interesting, roughly coinciding as it did, with restrictions which summarily curtailed its practice in its traditional context of Koho Anma. Kanpo doctors were not known for their promotion of manual therapy and acknowledgement by such an esteemed doctor must be regarded as an important recognition and one that would have been taken seriously. Genetsu Kagawa (1700–1777) was another well-known figure in this field. Working as a Haratori, specialising in obstetrics, during the same period as Yoshimasu, he made his own

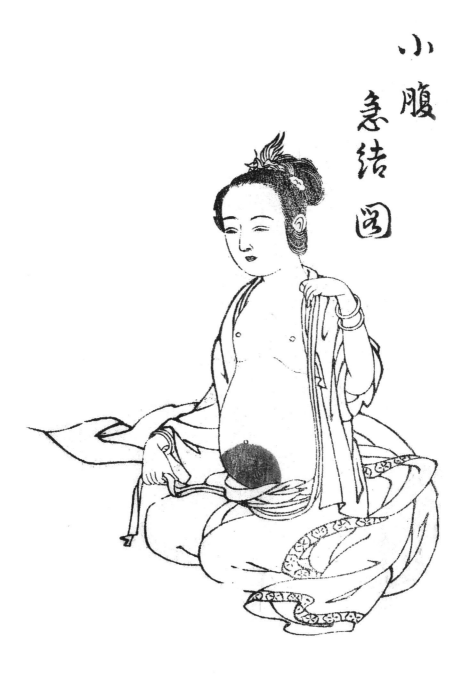

小腹急結図

Fuku-Shin from *Toho-Binran* by Todo Yoshimasu

investigations called the 'seven arts of obstetrics' which was a kind of Shiatsu that included hara diagnosis. When Western charts of anatomy became more widely available, his work was reassessed and many of his findings were confirmed. He overturned long-held and erroneous beliefs based on the Chinese systems of medicine, making great strides forward in his field.

In 1827, in another shift away from the Edo period's restrictions, Fusai Ota published *Anpuku Zukai* (*Illustrated Anpuku*), in which he said that this was important medicine that could be understood and performed by anyone and, as such, should not be controlled. Originally an Anma practitioner himself, Fusai Ota had become seriously ill and, finding no help in his own profession, set out to cure himself. Guided by insights thus gained, he asserted that the ever-growing emphasis on technique in Anma had replaced real expertise. Rather than enhance its professional status, as the Anma Association contended, it contributed to the demotion of their art, reducing its scope to physical stimulation. By contrast, Anpuku could not be classified as stimulation and demanded of the practitioner a more refined approach. Treating the hara could not be performed with the same style of touch used to relax muscles and, in a development that influenced later Shiatsu practitioners, called for deep, stationary pressure and a focused sensitivity. *Suiatsu* was the name that Fusai Ota gave to this method and his book is pointed to as the beginning of modern Shiatsu.

Thus, Anpuku, Koho Anma and Suiatsu all carry elements that later echoed in Shiatsu. But it was not until the twentieth century, with the growing influence of Western science in traditional medicine, combined with a renewed interest in natural medicine and the philosophy of health, that Shiatsu emerged to fill the gap left by Koho Anma, and caught the attention of a small band of idealistic and ambitious philosophers, doctors and manual therapists.

The Emergence of Shiatsu in Twentieth-Century Japan

By the twentieth century, Anma had been regulated again and practitioners were prohibited from working without an official licence. But it was not hard to circumvent the rules. Practitioners without it simply chose another name for what they did and carried on working. One such name was *Shiatsu*. Simply meaning a form of 'finger pressure', it could cover any number of methods but pointed to none in particular.

As the name gained usage, practitioners looked for commonality and started developing theory as the foundation for a new classification. In doing so, and in common with other manual therapists at the time, the new Shiatsu therapists turned to the massage traditions of the West for inspiration. Both fashionable and scientific in a world that increasingly looked to categories and measurement over the vagaries of quality, this underpinning lent the new method some professional credibility. But it was not until the 1919 publication of Tenpeki Tamai's *Shiatsu-Ho* (*Shiatsu Therapy*) that Shiatsu was really put on the map. Although it has not stood the test of time and is little used today, the book was a classic of early Shiatsu and an important milestone, putting together a theoretical foundation for the infant therapy with the skills of Anpuku diagnostics and focused manual technique.

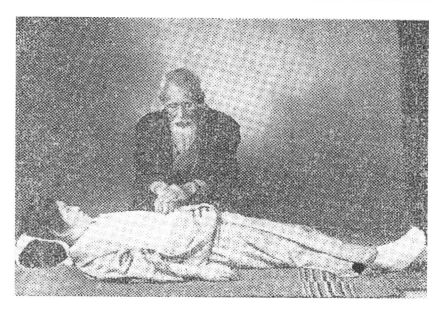

Tenpeki Tamai, the father of Shiatsu

A decade later, as Shiatsu was beginning to gain a following, it received a huge boost to its profile through the inclusion of some basic instructions in a new edition of a popular compendium of family health, known as *The Red Book*. By this time, Shiatsu was a name familiar to the Japanese public, with several books of theory and practice available.[21]

Compiled by a naval officer, Takichi Tsukuda, *The Red Book*[22] was published in its original form in 1925. It included remedies for all manner of ailments and a huge range of tips, recipes and techniques.

---

21 In the early Showa period (1926–1989) a book called *Shiatsutherapy* was published which mentioned several other works on Shiatsu, demonstrating that this new therapy was increasingly in the public arena. Such books include: Hirata, K. *Seitai and Shiatsu Therapy*; Tamai, T. (1919) *Shiatsu Therapy*; Takagi, R. *Takagi-Style Shiatsu*; Kuriyama, K. and Namikoshi, T. (1934) *Shiatsutherapy and Physiology*. Tokyo: Keibundo-syoten. Revised edition (with added dietary therapy) 1954.

22 *The Red Book* is a nickname for *The Know How of Practical Home Nursing* (1925) by Takichi Tsukuda (published by Tsukudamikizono-sya). The popular name derived from the book's distinctive red cover. It ran to 1615 editions and sold over 10 million copies in Japan. After the first edition of 1925 it went through many revisions. Prewar it was regarded as a necessity in Japanese homes and was a comprehensive compilation of folk remedies.

Although its target audience had originally been the limited world of naval families, it swiftly became a national bestseller and remained so until the 1960s. The revised edition of 1929 featured a supplementary section on folk medicine that included Shiatsu. Its detailed illustrations and descriptions of techniques and points for use with friends and family increased the growing interest in its professionalisation.

During this period the government made another attempt to control manual therapies. In a project that aimed to draw a clear line between Anma and the numerous other manual methods then available and establish a system of regulation, 300 therapies were investigated. This latest research was conducted by the police and the findings were published by Shigeyuki Ikematsu in 1939. Each therapy was put into one of five general categories: heat therapy, ray therapy, electrotherapy, massage and Shiatsu. The name 'Shiatsu' was used in this census because it was already in the public arena. Although the category did not refer to a clearly defined method, its inclusion evinced a growing awareness.

In these early years of the twentieth century, there were also some Shiatsu therapists who caught the attention of the public through well-publicised cures. One of these, Zentaro Koyama, gained celebrity for curing the Home Secretary of stomach cancer. His treatments involved very hard pressing and the account he gave of his Shiatsu was that it was *blood circulation therapy*. His high profile furthered its cause and augmented public demand.

Among the contemporaries of Tenpeki Tamai was another influential writer in the field, Sadakatsu Daikoku. Having researched many methods of natural health and written six books on traditional medicine, including Acupuncture and *Seitai*,[23] he concluded that manual therapy was the most potent and, in 1941, sought to revive Anpuku by reprinting Fusai Ota's nineteenth-century classic. The original had not been especially accessible and Sadakatsu Daikoku now added an extended introduction that brought Anpuku touch to the attention of Shiatsu practitioners and guided them in its use. Later, in 1964, Shiatsu practitioner Tadashi Izawa reinterpreted Sadakatsu Daikoku's work, making it still more comprehensible in his own

---

23   A form of movement therapy.

account, *Anpuku-Zukai and Shiatsutherapy*.[24] These practitioners were key figures, carrying the Shiatsu lineage that runs from Fusai Ota and Tenpeki Tamai through to Namikoshi, Masunaga and Kishi.

The growing public and professional interest in Shiatsu saw many therapists and theorists contributing to theory. But its close association with Anma, other manual therapies and natural medicine were connections that some more ambitious practitioners found problematic and there were moves to define it in separate terms that might elevate it from the problematic realm of subjectivity to that of science.

---

24 Izawa, T. (1964) *Anpuku and Shiatsutherapy*.

Post-War Shiatsu

From 1945 to 1952, in the aftermath of the Second World War, Japan was governed by a relatively benign Allied administration dominated by the United States. As part of its policy to rebuild Japan as a tame Western-style democracy, the administration banned non-licensed traditional medicine. Anma therapists were permitted to continue working, but anyone wanting to train after 1945 had to attend official massage school for two years which replaced the old five year apprenticeships. The proposed school system did not permit the flexibility that had made the apprenticeships workable for Shiatsu therapists who wanted to work with a licence, since the Anma licence was the only one available to them and they disliked the change.

In the light of this ruling, the Ministry of Health and Welfare approached universities throughout Japan for research input in clarifying the numerous therapies then on offer in scientific terms. Under the auspices of Dr Fujii, the physician in charge of investigating Shiatsu, the administration gave eight years' grace for researchers to come up with evidence that this method was, as they claimed, fundamentally different from Anma. The demand of the authorities did not reflect interest in the niceties of these distinctions but, rather, a wish to accurately codify licences in a common medical lexicon.

With some formidable characters among its early proponents, the research team put together to look into Shiatsu boasted talented practitioners alongside medical doctors and academics who, together, might do justice to the project. In Japan at that time, and in some respects even more so in recent times, doctors trained in the hard sciences were nonetheless interested in the traditional healing methods. So, while to Western readers, the presence of prominent medics and academics at the sharp end of defining and supporting what is characterised in the West as 'alternative therapy', cannot be seen in those terms in Japan since the same distinctions have never been made. Nonetheless, science was the dominant narrative through which Japanese medicine was perceived so, while it remained prominent, in practice it was undermined at its philosophical roots.

The task the researchers faced was far from straightforward, not least because the existence alongside each other of traditional and scientific medicine was rarely accompanied by an appreciation of the fundamental incongruities between them. Nonetheless, the team first had to agree upon a descriptive framework on which Shiatsu could be said to work in scientific terms. Dr Yoshio Daigyou, an author himself on physiology and hygiene, instructed the team in what was needed in the following terms (paraphrased):

> The requirement is to describe and prove satisfactory data on Shiatsu using language in which other people can understand the effects of it. However, Japanese medicine, in contrast with modern science, falls short of the mark in this. In this tradition, expertise finishes with a particular person's mastering of it. With their death, the means and method of explaining it to the next generation are lost.[25]

By which he pointed out that the problem with proving the efficacy of Shiatsu in scientific terms is that the art is practised by individual masters who teach their own students in close, personal transmission. The means of teaching it to the next generation dies with each master and it had, for centuries, defied theoretical expostulation. Thus, the task before the research team was arguably contradictory and certainly ambitious in trying to describe, in scientific language, something that could not conform to scientific definition. It highlighted the centuries-old tension between objective textual authority and subjective authority, individual transmission and structured school training. However, the team did not see this as a conflict so much as a challenge, assuming that rendering this manual art into a formal conceptual framework was one of translation rather than fundamental incompatibility.

---

25 Quoted from text provided by Kyoko Kishi to the authors, June 2010.

It was at this time that two great innovators in the field came into their own. Although Tenpeki Tamai first gave shape to Shiatsu, it was Tokujiro Namikoshi who requisitioned the name and made it famous for his home-grown style of manual therapy. Working alongside him, his student and colleague, the younger Shizuto Masunaga brought a strong academic background to the table along with his own training in Shiatsu. These two joined the team in addressing the task laid out by Daigyou.

In the first instance, practical experiments were conducted in which Anma was performed according to the formal principles laid out by the Ministry of Health and Welfare.[26] Shiatsu treatments were then given in equally controlled circumstances and, to the surprise of some investigators, produced quite different results.

Continuing in this manner, according to the formalities of established scientific methodology, the research team gathered and analysed an enormous amount of data on the effects of Shiatsu and strove to form the results into a coherent thesis. The conclusion they finally came to was, in brief, that Shiatsu decreased the activity of the sympathetic nervous system in the course of which the parasympathetic nervous system became predominant, so promoting a state of rest. Conversely, Anma was understood to stimulate the sympathetic nervous system and promote activity.

Thus the team agreed that Anma was effective as an adjustment before and after activity and was effective in supporting a fundamentally healthy state. Shiatsu, on the other hand, was more effective in addressing established illness; quietening the mind and body of the sick person to affect the condition at a deep level.

This explanation, couched in modern medical terms, lent Shiatsu a legitimacy and authority that helped develop its professional standing to act as a bridge between traditional healing and symptomatic medicine. Not only that, but the link with the parasympathetic nervous system boosted the confidence of Shiatsu practitioners in concretely demonstrating that their work was different from Anma, of specific medical value and could be discussed as such in clear terms.

---

26 In the textbook, *The Theory of Massage and Skill of Anma* (1976) by Katsusuke Serizawa, a blind professor, and Dr Seizaburo Sugi (published by Ishiyaku-syuppan).

The Anma Association was resistant to the attempt to separate Anma from Shiatsu since the already reduced profession feared slipping further in status without the inclusion of this swiftly developing method under its licence. Since Anma was known as a profession for blind people, they feared further social distinction. Determined to continue nonetheless, the researchers defined Shiatsu in fairly narrow terms that did not necessarily reflect the entirety of its practical reality or history but served the purpose of establishing it as a therapy in its own right, with its own principles, very efficiently.

In 1947 when the research teams were just being put together and much in the style of Japanese officialdom through the ages, a new set of regulations had reconfigured the existing categories of traditional medicine and had established licences for Anma, Acupuncture, Moxibustion and *Judo Kappo*.[27] In 1955, Shiatsu had gained a degree of recognition when the Anma licence was changed to include it, along with massage. But it was not until 1964 that they were finally able to operate under a named licence, much to Namikoshi's advantage since his college in Tokyo became the only institution that fulfilled the requirements needed for the national licence in Shiatsu.

The period of this research was a rich time for Shiatsu and a number of seminal books on what was then known as *Shiatsutherapy* were published. Initially, in 1954, Namikoshi and Dr Kinzo Kiriyama revised their 1934 book, *Shiatsutherapy and Physiology*,[28] to include dietary advice. This was followed by *Health and Hygiene*[29] in 1957, by one of the principal researchers, Dr Fusajiro Kato, who devoted half his book to Shiatsutherapy and specifically recommended its use for maintaining good relations with friends and family.

Following this, Kato worked with Masunaga on a more in-depth study that was closely linked to the government research. The result of this collaboration, *Principles of Shiatsutherapy*[30] in 1963, instantly became a principal textbook of the Japan Shiatsu College in Tokyo. It also served to formally establish the distinctions between Anma and

27 Judo Kappo is also known as Judo Seifuku or Bonesetting.
28 Kuriyama, K. and Namikoshi, T. (1934) *Shiatsutherapy and Physiology*. Tokyo: Keibundo-syoten. Revised edition (with added dietary therapy) 1954.
29 Kato, F. (1957) *Health and Hygiene*. Tokyo: Kunimitsu-syobo.
30 Kato, F. and Masunaga, S. (eds) (1968) *Principles of Shiatsutherapy*. Tokyo: Daiichi-syuppan.

Shiatsu and acted as the final report of the research team, ensuring its success in gaining recognition. Following swiftly on from this first success, Masunaga, this time working with Dr Hisayoshi Yamaguchi, published *The Clinical Practice of Shiatsu*[31] in 1965, a companion volume that joined the first as a core teaching text.

However, for some of the researchers, the project had not just been about gaining separate recognition for Shiatsu, but was part of a grander movement that aimed to relocate or return Eastern philosophy to the centre of all aspects of life, pointing to the home-grown combination of *Zen*, *Taoism* and *Shinto* as their inspiration. In promoting Shiatsu they were prompted by hope for a new age in which this account of the human condition and its idea of a 'natural' alleviation of suffering could be used to conduct all medical intervention towards a common end, bringing the ideal of harmonious life into a workable reality.

The scope of this thinking was far-reaching and, as is often the way with utopias, not successful in the first instance. But to understand the genesis of Shiatsu it must be seen, not as an isolated therapy trying to make its way in the world among other similar methods, but as philosophical rather than medical at base, and an aspect of this wider ideology.

As was perhaps inevitable in turning Shiatsu into a profession, the requirements of a transparent theory and the realities of practice were now in potential competition. Daigyou's statement of the problem for the government sponsored research had only been solved temporarily. For some members of the team the task of development and definition was only just beginning.

On the one hand, professional recognition and structured training aimed towards wide dissemination and could work only on a fairly basic theoretical framework. On the other, the actual practice of Shiatsu, learned through hands-on experience, depended upon the authority of the experienced practitioner, taught through one-to-one transmission. Manual therapy had always eluded formal description. While the researchers had been given the remit to explain Shiatsu in scientific terms, which they had achieved well enough to satisfy the

---

31 Yamaguchi, H. and Kato, F. with Masunaga, S. (eds) (1965) *The Clinical Practice of Shiatsu.* Tokyo: Daiichi-syuppan.

authorities, the process of investigation had in fact led them in an unexpected direction. During the period of research, they had found themselves moving away from the scientific model towards Eastern philosophy as a more satisfactory theory base. This was, perhaps, no surprise since Koho Anma, from which Shiatsu took so much of its inspiration, harked back to an age of medical apprenticeships and the prioritisation of subjective knowledge. But, as with all attempts to return to basics, it was also a political reformulation of 'tradition' as seen through the ideologically motivated eyes of progressives interested in restoring an idealised golden age.

Although the research of the 1940s to the 1960s represented a height of foment around Shiatsu that has never been matched, it really only served to put it on the map; it now qualified as legitimate Japanese medicine,[32] in what was supposed to be the first step in restoring manual therapy to its rightful place as equal, and even pre-eminent, among the other medical arts.

While Namikoshi went from success to success with his busy college and high public profile, Masunaga was not content to sit back and enjoy the achievements of the research team. Although persuaded that the explanation the team had arrived at was a good beginning, he was not satisfied that Shiatsu had yet attained its ideal form or that the theory was sufficiently developed. He spent the rest of his life developing basic Shiatsu practice and constructing an account premised on an Eastern philosophical ideal, trusting that this inherent tension would be resolved through enough application and the appropriate formal underpinning.

---

32 In 1957, *The Shiatsutherapy Reader* was published by T. Ogawa (Tokyo: Ido no Nihon-sya). This book attracted attention because the publisher was known for books on Acupuncture- and Moxibustion-related works and, in this book, is seen to be putting Shiatsu in the same category.

Tokujiro Namikoshi (1905–2000)

None was more successful under the Shiatsu banner in its early decades than Tokujiro Namikoshi. He began practising manual therapy as a child to ease his mother's crippling arthritis and discovered that steady pressure with his palms and thumbs relieved her pain and ultimately alleviated the condition altogether. He was quickly recognised as the possessor of a very special talent. But, though in demand, without an official licence he was limited in what he could do without interference from the authorities. To remedy this, and still only in his teens, he travelled to Tokyo to gain a licence in Anma.

When he returned to his family in Hokkaido, Namikoshi immediately set up a practice. Although naturally influenced by his Anma schooling, when he adopted the name Shiatsu for his approach after Tenpeki Tamai's example, he made a clear departure from that training and focused on the method that had grown out of his own experimentation and was closest to Anpuku. In 1925 he opened the Shiatsu Institute of Therapy in Hokkaido and, in 1940, the Japan Shiatsu Institute in Tokyo, which later became the Japan Shiatsu College, to disseminate his method.

Namikoshi was a well-known and much liked man. His broad, smiling face became a familiar sight on television for the regular slots in which he demonstrated and explained useful points for home remedies. A key figure in gaining official recognition for Shiatsu, his celebrity clientele did his cause no harm and he particularly delighted in telling stories about Marilyn Monroe. By this time, Shiatsu was an established therapy, but Japan was also becoming a modern state at a galloping pace; traditional therapies, with their pace and approach of former times, were not always appealing, so Namikoshi's 1967 book, *Three Minute Shiatsu*,[33] was well judged, perfectly suited to a world in which the *instant* was marketable and helped add to the growing number of enthusiasts. But it was his charm that clinched the deal and the public could not get enough of him.

Namikoshi was ambitious for Shiatsu, sharing some of the utopian hopes of many of his colleagues. His personal ambition extended, at one point, to standing for Parliament, although he was not in the end elected, and his close involvement in the research and licensing of Shiatsu and his establishment of the Japan Shiatsu College were key features of this wider vision. The institutional setting of the college called for straightforward theory and practice that could easily be replicated, and the definition of Shiatsu, now formalised, served it well enough in its primary aim of training people in a profession that would earn them a living. Shiatsu seemed set to be taken seriously as both a viable career and as a medical option.

Students of all ages and different backgrounds were admitted to the college through an interview and written examination, and given an education anchored primarily in Western anatomy and physiology, particularly 'pressure reflex theory'[34] and, secondarily, in general Kanpo. This was done with the aim of passing the state examinations in Shiatsu. Namikoshi saw little point in developing this theory further and regarded philosophical questions about cure, health and sickness as less important than practice. His focus was on the quality he called *touch with love* from which, he said, the spring of life would flow when properly employed.

His own treatments were by all accounts exceptional but this skill could not be passed on to any but the few who were close to him requiring, as it did, years of practice to master the subtleties. In a simplification of his personal approach, his college taught a set routine that became Namikoshi-style Shiatsu. The skill of understanding the precise effect of every point, through touch and

---

33 Namikoshi, T. (1967) *Three Minute Shiatsu*. Tokyo: Jitsugyo no Nihon-sya.
34 The effect of pressure on points on the body to the organs.

'sight'[35] that characterised Namikoshi's own Shiatsu, was harder to achieve and, in attempting to copy that style his disciples imitated the outer form and performed it more strongly than he did in a fast, one-point pressure technique. Thus, in the college setting, Namikoshi's principle of holding focused pressure was largely lost. But the training was popular and fitted the modern idea of professionalisation that advocated quick solutions and a professional demeanour as key to the commodification of Shiatsu.

Namikoshi-style Shiatsu is known in Japan, and by his disciples, as definitive; his was the only Shiatsu college, so debates that arise in the West between different private Shiatsu schools are not seen in Japan. He rode the wave of popular interest and augmented it, bringing in a professional format that has also gained some popularity in Europe and North America where its formal routine can fairly easily be promulgated.

However, Shiatsu existed before Namikoshi. While he gave it an important boost and personally influenced many teachers through the quality of his touch and presence, others have built on their common foundations and developed the work in different ways.

One such man was Shizuto Masunaga. His personal mission to explain and convey the full dimensions of Shiatsu to university standard opened the work to a wider audience. His approach was more in tune with the interests and direction of the twenty-first century than those who came before and it is Masunaga whom many in the West point to as their exemplar. It is his character of innovation and articulation that continues to inspire.

---

35 By 'sight' he meant that the mind opens into the fingertips.

Shizuto Masunaga
(1925–1981)

In 1957, the year that Namikoshi opened the Japan Shiatsu College in Tokyo, Shizuto Masunaga was among the first to enrol, graduating in 1959. He was already an experienced therapist, having been introduced to Shiatsu by his mother, Shizuka Masunaga. She had studied under Tenpeki Tamai and, indefatigable in her pursuit of understanding, continued to attend workshops with a number of well-known teachers. Believing that it represented a noble and worthy profession, she resolved that one of her three sons must be trained in the art and took them with her on workshops with this in mind. Initially just an observer, by the age of 13 Masunaga was gaining hands-on experience with some of the greatest teachers of the age, including masters Sadakatsu Daikoku, Zentaro Koyama and Major General Sugiyama.

A retired military man, Sugiyama was a master practising his own style of Shiatsu. At only 15, Shizuka Masunaga took her son to him, asking that Sugiyama admit him as a student. Understandably doubtful that a young boy could have the gravity to perform treatment with the proper level of professionalism, he was finally persuaded that Masunaga had the correct attitude and agreed to do so.

Masunaga, however, was also academically gifted and, perhaps placed in the world of manual therapy against his natural inclinations, quickly applied his powerful analytical skills to the art in what became a lifelong interest. Later attending the prestigious Kyoto University where he studied psychology, he was expected by his tutors there to pursue the career in the Academy that seemed to fit his talents so well. But, although the path he chose for himself in articulating Shiatsu was academic in important respects, it remained outside the university sector until the last years of his life.

Although he had initially thought his mother's profession problematically unscientific, Masunaga found himself won over by its effectiveness and simple human appeal and channelled his energy into researching its roots in the belief that it represented a revolutionary approach to medicine that must find a place alongside its more illustrious cousins in the old medical arts.

With his unusual combination of intellectual and practical training, Masunaga was perfectly suited to join the researchers engaged in the project to define Shiatsu for official ratification. It served his own purposes exactly and many of the published results can be attributed to him, though little carried his name. But when the licence was finally granted, he did not regard the project as complete. While Shiatsu now had some potential as an academic subject, the established theory offered a limited explanation that did not touch on the philosophy which he believed more accurately represented its underpinnings.

Masunaga continued his research as a teacher at Namikoshi's college from 1959 to 1969. His classes were regularly packed and he drew on his wide interests to teach a broad curriculum that included clinical psychology and the philosophy of both East and West. His energy for exposition and development made him an exciting teacher. But his style was not to everyone's taste and deviated from the standard college line. Some of his colleagues complained about his controversial combinations of subjects which, in turn, offended him and prompted his departure from the college in 1969, despite the good personal relationship he always enjoyed with Namikoshi. Since he had set up his own, postgraduate, establishment the year before, removing there was, in any case, an obvious step.

The name that Masunaga chose for his institute, *Iokai*, was also a statement of his personal manifesto. Its elements stand for: *I* – medicine, *O* – king and *Kai* – association, reflecting his belief that Shiatsu was the ultimate medicine. A private institute, it was not a licence-awarding college but a largely postgraduate institution, the majority of the disciples[36] having already gained a qualification, either in Shiatsu or another recognised therapy.

Having given a great deal of thought to how it should be taught, his vision was that teaching would take place using a small tutorial format that mimicked the earlier apprentice system and moved away from the trend towards large institutions and classes. It was a template intended to maintain quality while keeping the art available, embracing the best of both worlds.

In fact this ideal was never properly realised. Already a well-known, highly respected and even awe-inspiring figure, small class teaching was not Masunaga's style or preference and he rarely welcomed the intimacy of conversation with students, remaining a reserved and enigmatic figure to most.

Indeed, many disciples found it hard to understand what Masunaga said and complained that he spoke in Zen-style *koans* – unanswerable riddles that left them with a sense that something precious lay hidden in his words if only they could understand. Although this added considerably to his aura of authority and mystique, some longed for simpler explanations. Ironically, although the provision of an accessible theory was his life's focus, few students had the academic background or interest to meet him in this and he remained an isolated figure.

In the work of one contemporary, however, he found an important ally. Although they probably never met, Kurakichi Hirata was a contemporary of Masunaga's at Kyoto University and, like him, combined academic excellence with an interest in the practical philosophy of healing and the harmonious life. Although he died in the Second World War at the age of 44, he had already contributed several volumes to the field. Since any question about the *good life* must engage with a diagnosis of our present condition, the solution is never far from some notion of medicine and Hirata's work[37] included

---

36 'Disciple' is a more appropriate term than 'student' for a Japanese student and for Masunaga's school and style of teaching.

37 Initially a student of philosophy, Kurakichi Hirata's enquiries had led him to the study of Western medicine. But in this training he found himself again asking the fundamental philosophical questions he had started with. This time he found the most satisfactory answers were to be found in traditional healing, so much so that he gave up his medical degree shortly before graduation. In Hirata's vision of medical help, a prerequisite was

proposals for a healing model very much in line with Masunaga's own project of developing the ideal Shiatsu.

In the 1930s, when Hirata was writing, there were numerous manual therapies available, many of which were influenced by the scientific project of demystifying the body. Since this had been the official medical model since the mid-nineteenth century, therapists in the old medical arts sought to use this theory as a base to explain their own methods. However, that was a project that both Masunaga and Hirata saw as fundamentally flawed in joining together approaches that were founded on incompatible precepts.

In developing manual therapies up to university standard, both men proposed that Eastern philosophy, rather than science, must serve as their common foundation. As long as these fundamentals were agreed, they argued, people could then add whatever they liked, including Western ideas, if they served the core ideology.

Hirata was known to have performed manual therapy in accord with his account of theory but, while it sounds like Masunaga's Shiatsu in some respects, details of his treatments are not extant; although some of his principles, such as his 'twelve zones', are still used in some Japanese therapies. For Masunaga, the discovery of a like-minded soul served as confirmation that he was on the right track and gave force to his project of explaining and teaching Shiatsu as both the heart and pinnacle of medicine.

---

that the sick person sincerely accepts their pain, while the helper spontaneously applies a 'formal stimulus'. The helper's observation is key in this scenario. If it is clear, then they will perceive the centre of the sickness and pain in conjunction with performing a spontaneous act of stimulation. This treatment was ideal in that it combined the patient's own awareness and conscious participation with direct, spontaneous action precisely in tune with the expression of disease. In this way, the person could be said to have cured themselves. In describing self-cure, he advocated looking straight at your pain, with palms joined together for focus, perceive its emotional strength and in so doing, drawn this out. Pain is thus transformed into joy and the problem purified in the most satisfactory manner.

In his 1932 *Medical Examination Encyclopaedia* (published by Kimura-syobo), Hirata discussed the nature of illness and a model of the medical ideal. In framing the proper attitude for medical intervention, he asserted that what the sick person is looking for is not so much a complex pathology of the disease, but practical help. Technique, he stated, is relatively straightforward and can be learned in one day with enough determination; but this is not medicine either. Manual therapy was his ideal and his aim was to educate people, mainly in the home, so that friends and family could perform treatments both effectively and economically.

While theory was a major preoccupation for Masunaga, he was alive to the need to align it with best practice. Practice, of course, varied with each practitioner, reflecting personal influences and tendencies; Namikoshi's Shiatsu was in the *ho-ho* style, naming the character of soft touch he employed, while Masunaga himself used stronger pressure, the *sya-ho* method. But whatever the differences of personal approach might be, Masunaga wished to develop a teaching form through which every student could understand the basics of effective performance. In this teaching model, personal talent and style was, if anything, something of a spanner in the works.

The Shiatsu taught at Namikoshi's college had moved away from his quality of touch to reflect the needs of a busy institution. Students were taught to work with palms and thumbs along a series of prescribed points or *tsubos*. Far from Namikoshi's example, it could be an uncomfortable experience for the patient. Masunaga sought to improve this one-point pressure with a two-handed method that prioritised the comfort of both parties. With one hand 'listening', the therapist's field of awareness and sensitivity was said to increase. With this 'supported pressure', patient and practitioner were comfortably stabilised and two hands were experienced as unified contact since two points held on the same *meridian* establish an echo.

While this two-handed technique has formed the focus for much of the teaching of Masunaga's Shiatsu since then, it was developed to facilitate the heart of Masunaga's Shiatsu, *sesshin*.[38] His research into the principles of traditional medicine, and manual therapy in particular, led him to an understanding of the essence of Eastern, specifically Japanese, diagnostics that required an holistic approach that he believed had been reduced or lost in traditional medicine. Taking a cue from Koho Anma and its development of Anpuku as an exemplar, he sought to reinvigorate traditional diagnostics with Shiatsu at its centre. Sesshin, a term used in Acupuncture diagnosis, had to be understood anew. In establishing it in his own terms as a core practice and model, he hoped to be able to teach Shiatsu more effectively.

---

38 Sesshin is one of the four diagnostic skills of Kanpo.

In time, Masunaga moved through several subject areas to find a suitable language to articulate Shiatsu, although sesshin remained at its centre and, by 1964, he had returned to psychology and psychotherapeutic theory as a possible framework.

Psychology was a subject close to Masunaga's heart, but, as an addition to Shiatsu, it was a departure from accepted approaches and regarded by traditional therapists as a step too far. Nonetheless, he researched this field, finding in the work of Carl Rogers[39] and his idea of *unconditional positive regard*, a theory that compared well with his own idea that successful therapy rested primarily on the attitude and presence of the therapist. In Japanese philosophy, however, mind and body cannot be regarded as separable. Since the traditional doctor must understand the patient in every dimension in order to perform medicine effectively, the division of the psychological into a separate sphere was not only incomprehensible, but also scandalous to suggest. In any case, Masunaga soon rejected psychology as an overarching theory for Shiatsu, although its influence on his work remained.

The traditional medical systems of China represented a more comprehensive possibility for him as a source of theory, and a more lasting one and, by the late 1960s after his departure from the Japan Shiatsu College, he was researching it in earnest.

While Chinese medicine informed the early development of medicine in Japan, it must now be seen through the filter of hundreds of years of local use and development. A Western scholar researching the Chinese classics without this perspective cannot replicate the conclusions that Masunaga, a master and proponent of *Japanese* medicine and philosophy, saw and made use of in developing Shiatsu. This is especially so if the Chinese medicine studied is TCM, standardised with a specific ideological agenda by the communist regime in the 1950s.

Since Chinese medical theory was developed in the very different practice of Acupuncture, his attempt to join it with Shiatsu was controversial and he entered into some fierce debates with the

---

39 Carl Rogers was one of the founding fathers of the humanistic approach to psychology and client-centred therapy.

professional Acupuncture association over his deployment of it for his own purposes.

Sesshin was not the only theoretical concept he made use of: traditional Chinese and traditional Japanese medicine employed a meridian theory which Masunaga thought could be helpful in describing the experience of Shiatsu for teaching purposes. Primarily from the Acupuncture tradition but also finding expression in Anma, it was new to Shiatsu and, like other elements of Chinese medical practice, not a straight transplant. Masunaga understood that meridian philosophy would need to find a specifically Shiatsu-orientated expression to be incorporated into his work. He worked at this for years and continued to fine-tune his account to the end of his life, with a version of sesshin and meridian philosophy that extended far beyond the purview of its inspiration. The addition of meridian maps and philosophy to Shiatsu appealed to many who practised it in his name but his disciples, both Eastern and Western, have not always appreciated is purpose. Western students embraced it in a vacuum, without the grounding experience of practical training and, particularly in the West, Chinese medicine has been put at the centre of Masunaga's Shiatsu and informs many modern interpretations of his work, resulting in an emphasis and misunderstandings that persist to this day.

Useful or not, Chinese medical theory was not to the taste of all his disciples, but nor was it core teaching in the early days. Iokai members were impressed, time and again, with the far more insistent instruction to perform sesshin, learning through subjective feeling. When Masunaga later tried to fit his theories onto Shiatsu practice, some disciples found the work less interesting and, disliking his new and less flexible approach, gradually moved away.

Although sometimes controversial, many therapists attended Masunaga's Iokai workshops in the 1970s and accord him great respect to this day. His influence outside Japan, however, while also considerable, has been problematic.

The Iokai initially attracted only Japanese members but over the years, as word of Shiatsu reached interested ears abroad, foreigners began knocking on the door asking for instruction. Since they did not need to be certified in Japan in order to practise in their homelands, many came straight to the Iokai rather than first applying for Namikoshi's official training. However, their lack of experience was a handicap since disciples at Masunaga's institute practised on members of the public. Foreigners without the necessary licence could not do so and consequently did not gain the experience and tutoring that the public clinics offered, thereby missing essential elements of the programme. On top of this, for his own reasons, Masunaga was not especially interested in teaching foreigners and for the most part avoided them. However, they were permitted to participate in short courses with weekly classes for set periods, through several levels. Reflecting the differences, the certificate awarded to these members bore a separate numbering system from that given to natives.

Although many Westerners took a taste of his Shiatsu home with them, it was in an attenuated form. Even those for whom the desire to learn was sincere and persistent were rarely afforded the opportunity of much personal contact or mentoring. An art that was acknowledged by Masunaga as needing at least some personal transmission for effective teaching and learning was largely denied to foreigners.

Western Shiatsu has suffered from the limited teaching available as those foreigners who did study with him were unable to pass it on with fidelity to the original. While some of the responsibility for this can be laid at Masunaga's feet, the situation was, perhaps more fairly, an accurate reflection of the limited possibilities of the era. Since Masunaga's approach was also too difficult for most of his native disciples to fully grasp, the task was an impossible one for foreigners who also had to contend with language and cultural hurdles.

Another feature of the uncertain export of Masunaga's Shiatsu to the West is the notable failure of Shiatsu as an international body to translate most of his writings into the vernacular of the countries that adopted it. The most obvious reason for this is that manual therapy rarely attracts those whose interest lies equally in intellectual exposition and sensitivity of touch. On top of this, translations require exemplary facility with languages to render texts that can be difficult even for a native speaker into a second language. It remains a woeful and bewildering omission nonetheless.

The major exception to this was Wataru Ohashi's 1977 translation of Masunaga's book, *Shiatsu*, into English under the title *Zen Shiatsu*.[40] A literature graduate educated in the United States but Japanese by birth, he, and his then assistant, Japanese-American Pauline Sasaki, were better suited than most to make the attempt.

Having emigrated to the United States in the 1960s, Ohashi became passionately interested in the medicine of his homeland and embarked on extensive research, ordering a great many books on the subject from Japan. Coming across Masunaga's writing, he entered into correspondence with him before travelling to Japan, later inviting the master to teach workshops in North America where he made a lasting impact.

On its own, *Zen Shiatsu* is just a fragment of a lifetime's work in Shiatsu. But, for most Western students, it is the only original text available to them. Without it, it is hard to say whether Shiatsu would have gained a foothold in the West, but its disproportionate influence has been problematic. It has not benefited from the expositionary presence of its author and is stranded outside its cultural and philosophical context without even the distinction of being Masunaga's seminal work.

Masunaga died young, with his project far from complete. Many of the theories he had developed and modified to explain Shiatsu, he had rejected by the time of his death but, up to the end, he was full of fresh ideas and seemed on the verge of a whole new approach. Yet his aim of raising Shiatsu to university level to stand alongside its better known counterparts as an accepted element of Japanese medicine, as Koho Anma had so long before, finally found some success. Just two years before he died, Masunaga was appointed professor at the Institute of Oriental Medical Research at the Kitazato University in Tokyo,[41]

---

40 Masunaga, S. with Ohashi, W. (1977) *Zen Shiatsu*. New York and Tokyo: Japan Publications.

41 The Foundation for Oriental Medical Research was established following the influence of Dr Taro Takemi, who was a highly influential doctor and head of the medicine medical association in the 1970s. Although a medic with a great deal at stake in promoting Western medicine, he developed an interest in Kanpo and asserted the importance of researching and developing it. His interest could not be ignored and, still today, some of the medical training in Japan offer modules on traditional medicine although they are not studied on their own terms but through the philosophical model of science.

fulfilling a lifetime's ambition and representing an acknowledgement from the highest echelons of the medical profession of the value of the Eastern approach.[42] But the victory was short-lived and, by the time of his death, Shiatsu had not been sufficiently established in that institution to outlive him and no successor to the post was appointed.

Masunaga's legacy has been as substantial as it has been misunderstood. While several innovators in the West and Japan have attempted to finish his project in his stead, without a clear understanding of the basics of his work or direction from the master, this has been a haphazard project.

Central to his work was the idea that, unless skill in manual treatment is prioritised, the essence of Eastern medicine cannot be maintained. For this reason, it is vital for Acupuncture and Moxibustion, as well as Shiatsu, to re-establish the priority of sesshin, one of the four pillars of diagnostics in Kanpo. As the conclusive factor of *syo diagnosis*,[43] it cannot be separated from treatment. While establishing this point was central to his work, it is not well understood in Japan and did not translate to Western Shiatsu, either in theory or practice.

But Masunaga's story does not end there. His top student and assistant for ten crucial years in the golden days of the Iokai, Akinobu Kishi has carried the spirit of his teaching into the new millennium. He has taught in Japan, Europe and North America for decades, first as Masunaga's disciple and scion and then on his own. A traditionalist and dissenter in equal parts, he is the perfect bridge between Masunaga's ideal and its practical application. Able to span the cultural mores of East and West, he not only explains his teacher's Shiatsu from the unique vantage point of the trusted intimate and acolyte, but has also developed Masunaga's ideal in the cauldron of cross-cultural connections and brings its heart, intact, to an international audience.

---

42   See Appendix II.

43   See Part II, In Conversation: Shiatsu for details of syo diagnosis.

Akinobu Kishi (born 1949)

Akinobu Kishi was introduced to manual therapy at an early age. His father, a businessman in the family company, had practised *Judo*[44] from childhood and was a local champion and seventh dan.[45] Before the Second World War it had been common for men to engage in martial arts training for well-being and as *Do*,[46] and Kishi himself practised *Karate*[47] as a child. Post-war, while this custom continued in a reduced way, the traditional patterns of life in Japan that had been slipping since the nineteenth century now mostly gave way and martial arts became more closely associated with sporting activities than with Do, as increasing emphasis was placed on career and success. But the old ways did not abruptly die in all households. Since injury was an accepted part of the art, many martial artists combined it with expertise in healing. Kishi's father augmented his natural talent through the study of Judo Kappo, a form of physiotherapy combining Western techniques with traditional massage and Bonesetting. Kishi observed his father's healing methods with interest and was encouraged to copy, practising on family and friends for pocket money.

Kishi's mother also had manual skills, both in massage and kimono making. As a schoolgirl, massage was offered as a subject for girls to prepare them for tending to the health of their future

---

44 Judo is a Japanese martial art.
45 Dan grades are a Japanese system of levels. Seventh dan is a very high level of achievement.
46 *Do* or *Way* is a Zen practice in which the traditional arts are studied as a path to wisdom and, ultimately, liberation.
47 Karate is a Japanese martial art.

families. So Kishi inherited talents from both parents and his interests set him a little apart from his contemporaries. But despite his hobbies, deeply rooted in the traditions of his culture as they were, he never felt entirely at home in Japanese society and longed to see the world, a desire fuelled by his uncle, a ship's doctor, whose tales of exotic lands fascinated the young boy.

Nonetheless, in 1968, putting therapy aside as an unsuitable career option in the judgement of his family, Kishi travelled south to the Tokyo Agricultural University to embark on a degree in landscape architecture. His interest in healing was deeply ingrained, however, and now a relatively free agent, he saw no reason not to pursue it on the side. By this time Namikoshi was a television celebrity and Shiatsu was enjoying huge popularity, so the Japan Shiatsu College was an obvious draw and he signed up for a workshop as soon as he could.

With ten years of home tutoring and practice behind him, Kishi was already an accomplished amateur having started his career in much the same way, and at much the same age, as the master himself. Although it was a short workshop, at which Namikoshi made only brief appearances, the famous man recognised Kishi's talent and offered him a much sought after studentship. Such an opening could not be taken lightly with 20 students competing for every place and, like Kishi, many of those accepted already had some experience through family apprenticeships.

Although Kishi's natural talent and facility had been informed by his parents' instruction and his own experimentation, like many masters over the years, his development was also fuelled by personal troubles that he had a keen interest in resolving.

Plagued from his early years by a fairly minor but uncomfortable complaint that did not respond to any of the usual remedies, school had represented a particular torture in requiring the young boy to sit still for hours on end. His persistent discomfort was a constant distraction and, instead of paying attention to lessons, Kishi turned his gaze inward in an unintended, but no less powerful, exploration of pain. One side effect of this, aside from an unimpressive academic record, was that his sensitivity to and understanding of body and mind was uncommonly well developed.

On top of his physical troubles, Kishi also found it awkward to communicate in ordinary social interaction. The only relationship in which he found empathic interaction natural and comfortable was manual contact. So Shiatsu was more than an interesting hobby for him. It represented, not only his most obvious natural talent and interest, but also a lifeline of human contact and the means of investigation through which he might cure his own problems.

By the time he met Namikoshi, the certainty Kishi felt in his own touch preceded anything he could be taught in a training which could only augment the existing authority of his treatments. But Kishi was impressed by Namikoshi's skill and the following year enrolled at the college alongside his university studies.

During his first year at Namikoshi's college, Kishi met the charismatic Masunaga and attended the clinical psychology and Eastern philosophy classes that he taught. Kyo/jitsu instruction was reserved for more experienced students; but Kishi was so keen that he paid little heed to formalities and joined the senior students who eagerly squeezed into Masunaga's packed classes.

When Masunaga left, Kishi had no intention of severing the tentative connection and immediately added classes at the Iokai to his schedule; he was fortunate to be accepted since he had not yet gained his licence. There, as was expected of all disciples, he dedicated himself to practice and kept his head down. As was also usual, the principal paid no obvious attention to him and Kishi merely dreamed of being singled out. As testament to his evident talent, he had not been attending classes for long when Masunaga asked him to perform a treatment. Awestruck, but delighted to have been recognised, Kishi did what he was told in what was the beginning of a close, ten-year apprenticeship.

Since Masunaga preferred lecturing to performing Shiatsu in front of classes, he was happy to find an assistant whose practical abilities reflected the principles he espoused. Having noticed the quality of Kishi's work and the understanding he evinced in his clinical practice, Masunaga regularly called on him to demonstrate while he addressed classes.

In contrast to Masunaga's hard technique that was painful to receive, Kishi's touch was uncommonly light and gentle, so the choice was an interesting one for Masunaga since their styles seemed, on the face of it, to be so different. But the two men worked well together and Kishi adored his teacher, hungrily absorbing everything the close connection afforded.

Of old, a good apprentice in the traditional Japanese arts was expected to observe and absorb in silence unless prompted by the master, who was trusted to know the right moment for the next stage of an acolyte's development. The Zen canon is littered with stories of greenhorn disciples asking impatient questions, only to be shown the error of their ways and the wisdom of obedient compliance. Question asking and initiative does not have a place in this situation and Masunaga certainly conformed to this model in the behaviour he expected of his disciples.

However, Kishi had never been a typical student and, having felt out of place for so long, he was finally in his element and full of queries. As such, he was a source of occasional annoyance to Masunaga, not only because he presumed to ask in the first place, but also because of the seemingly naive and fundamental nature of questions that put the teacher on his mettle. No one else wanted to risk displeasure by posing basic enquiries so fellow disciples, struggling with the same difficult demands that Masunaga made of all of them, were grateful that Kishi would put himself on the line to do so. Their teacher, although irritated at times and brusque in his responses, usually took his contributions seriously and their relationship was intimate and lively.

During this time, while Kishi was still barely in his twenties, he took leave from his commitments at home to embark on the first step in his career as an international practitioner and teacher. From early childhood Kishi had nursed a desire to travel to Europe, and France in particular. First smothered in the misery of his school days and then in the intense and restrictive atmospheres of his studies, he was bursting to break out for the romantic lure of Paris. Already an advanced student, having learned Masunaga's Shiatsu in only two years of close contact and already coming up against its limits, his teachers supported this step.

In 1971, speaking limited English and no French, he made the journey overland with just $500 in his pocket, the maximum then permitted when travelling through the USSR. Arriving in the city by train, he stepped straight into the middle of Paris with just a name and address with which to find his way.

Through connections at Namikoshi's college he had been offered space at a podiatry clinic before his departure and now made his way there, deeply relieved when he finally found his sponsors after the long journey.

Perhaps due to the language limitations of both parties, Kishi had failed to appreciate that he would be working at a foot clinic when he had accepted the invitation and was quietly surprised to discover the truth. But, grateful for the opportunity nonetheless and confident and flexible in his skills, he slotted into the clinic schedule and instantly became the darling of the chic female clientele. While this may have had something to do with his good looks and exotic appeal, he also impressed patients and colleagues with his unquestionable skill. They needed little persuasion of the value of moving from feet to whole body treatments and, with a steady stream of happy patients, in just a short time Kishi was setting up practices of his own in both Paris and Switzerland.

It was an interesting time to be in Western Europe; the cultural revolution that had swept the Western world from the late 1950s through to the early 1970s had brought in its wake a huge interest in alternative philosophies and a rejection of mainstream approaches to health and well-being. While many of these ideas had been explored by a few intellectuals and explorers over the previous few hundred years, for the first time, leisure time, education and communications were in place for dissemination on a larger scale. Riding this wave, Kishi was one of a small number of Easterners practising and teaching in the West whose views on life and health were embraced by those thirsty for alternatives. Welcomed into the homes and lives of patients and his growing body of disciples, Kishi was both amused and astonished at the attitudes he encountered, so different from those he had known from birth, but found many aspects of European life liberating. Having grown up under the restrictions of post-war Japan in a traditional family and then in the long shadows of his famous teachers, post-1968 Paris[48] was a heady place for him. He loved the personal and professional freedom he found there and was loved in return.

Kishi's first sojourn in Europe lasted 18 months before, in 1973, he reluctantly headed back to Tokyo to complete his degree. However, this was only the start of a long relationship with Europe where he later returned for several years at a time, living in Hamburg, Brussels and Munich in the 1980s.

Finally gaining his degree in 1974, Kishi did not retrace his steps to Europe immediately but travelled to Hawaii, a favourite destination of his compatriots. With apparently tireless energy he set up a practice once more and seemed unstoppable. The certainty in his hands transmitted itself to his ever growing number of patients and he thrived in every respect, briefly considering permanent immigration to the United States.

For Kishi, this period of his life was one of extremes. While he would spend hours in Shinto practice and seeing patients, this was interspersed with equally intense, hedonistic trips to Las Vegas. But, despite his business interests in Hawaii, Kishi never cut his ties with Japan and kept up his close relationship with Masunaga. The year 1974 saw them working together at the Korean Shiatsu Congress in the familiar roles of Kishi demonstrating with Masunaga lecturing. At the following year's Congress, when Masunaga suggested that it was time for his disciple to teach a workshop on his own approach, the topic Kishi chose was *The Principles of Shiatsu and Empathic Touch.*

In 1977, Kishi finally returned to Japan – a homecoming that marked another difficult decision in his life, since it meant leaving behind a successful practice again and the freedoms he so enjoyed. He went back, however, because he had failed one of the Hawaii State examinations required to continue working there as a therapist. Since he had little interest in medical law at the best of times and had already failed the exam twice, Kishi elected to take this as a prompt to return home.

---

48 There had been a great deal of left-wing inspired unrest, including a general strike and student agitations and sit-ins campaigning for social reform.

Returning to Japan always held its attractions and it was an important reconnection. During these years he had travelled back and forth between the United States and Japan and was always in close contact with the Iokai and in conversation with Masunaga. In going home, he looked forward to more regular contact.

However, although the relationship with Masunaga always remained one of deep respect, an end was in sight. In 1978–1979, he accompanied the mission of the Japanese Trade Federation round the world as one of their personal therapists. The delegates were among the top businesspeople in Japan and the tour was a major diplomatic and financial strategy for the Japanese government in building good relations and promoting trade. Traditional medicine was taken seriously at all levels of Japanese society as an important facet of healthcare, so to be invited to accompany these captains of industry was a well-paid honour. Yet, despite this acknowledgement and Kishi's appreciation of the good company and first class travel, the pinnacle of his success also marked the beginning of the end.

Before the trip, the stream of happy patients through his door had seemed unstoppable; he was doing so well that he had been able to buy himself a house in the expensive city of Tokyo. But, although his patients could hardly get enough of him and he now had a celebrity clientele of his own, this was in stark contrast to his own exhaustion and doubts. He began to wonder whether what he was seeing in his patients were any more than superficial changes while the underlying causes of their ill-health remained untouched. Whatever may have been the reality as far as his patients were concerned, Kishi could not deny that he had stagnated in his own development and this was not a situation he could continue to tolerate.

Returning home from the Trade Federation trip, he finally came to a halt and turned his attention to his own condition. Unable to find the integrity in his work that he wanted, he stopped seeing patients completely and, still only 29, Kishi fell into a profound depression. At this point he became interested in the Shinran sect,[49] joining the Shinran Society. Through this he came into contact with Shinto

---

49 Shinran (1173–1263) was a Japanese Buddhist monk and founder of what became the Jodo Shinshu sect.

mediums and his path of self-examination was set. Determined to examine the roots of his trouble, he surrendered himself to meditation and ritual Shinto purification. Some of this time was spent in the mountains near Kyoto meditating and chanting at an ancient shrine, sometimes staying in the forest through the night. He continued even during the harsh winter months, despite Shinto shrines being largely open to the elements and, in order to perform the ritual purification of *misogi* in the nearby mountain river, had to break ice to pour the frigid water on the crown of his head.

Back in Tokyo his meditations brought powerful and terrifying visions. Alone in his house, the crisis came to climax in three days of spontaneous movement that he later learned to call *katsugen*,[50] as years of suppressions and toxins found expression.

Obeying his instincts in the absence of any instruction in katsugen, he resolved to follow the feeling to its end and, surrendering to movement that rearranged his body and mind, Kishi's senses were sharpened and his mind cleared. When serenity finally found him, he was reborn.

Katsugen spontaneous movement is well documented in Shinto texts under different names,[51] such as *furube* (shaking) and *reido* (soul work). It is an important aspect of the clarifying required to lead a 'shining' or clear life. It was freshly named *katsugen undo*, within the broader discipline of Seitai, by Haruchika Noguchi[52] to separate it from its religious roots as categorically secular. Other forms of Seitai existed before and after Noguchi, and his use of katsugen was the mark of his own style. Despite being steeped in the practices of his homeland, however, katsugen was new to Kishi under any name. His lineage found him in any case and, in rediscovering it for himself he understood its value at a molecular level, later researching and discovering Noguchi's Seitai in particular, which was devoted to its cultivation for self-healing and development.

---

50 Katsugen is a regenerating movement.

51 Movement is known and encouraged in some Shinto practices and is related to norito (Shinto) recitation.

52 Noguchi (1911–1976) founded the Seitai Society and is known in Japan as an authority on ki.

But although Seitai was known to earlier proponents of Shiatsu, Masunaga had rejected it for professional and pedagogic reasons. He saw Noguchi's work as an expression of personal talent, so unsuitable for a formal teaching environment that called for uniformity.

Kishi's profound personal experience of katsugen, however, struck at the very root of his being, both illuminating and transforming him. His mind/body was altered and one of the first effects was that the haemorrhoids that had beset him from childhood were finally cured. A physical manifestation of the fundamental change that had taken place, the dramatic and instantaneous manner of this alteration reset his understanding of healing work at its very heart. Because it contained the genesis of his rebirth as well as a fresh approach to Shiatsu, it was finally he who was able to bring katsugen and Shiatsu together in a dynamic therapeutic practice.

Following his transformative experience, Kishi experienced phenomena common to awakening. Initially reluctant to see any patients, they nonetheless continued calling to make appointments and he discovered that he could treat people via the telephone, or even from photographs, with great success. Although his new powers were interesting, earning awed respect from patients and lending him the air of an impresario, he felt uncomfortable using them and dismissed his supernatural powers as party tricks, turning his attention back to straightforward sessions as soon as he was in a state of mind to receive patients again. But he went back to his work with completely new eyes.

The insight that came with his explosion into movement marked not only the beginning of a resolution to Kishi's immediate crisis but also the end of his relationship with Masunaga. This had been some time in coming. Despite Masunaga's ideal of teaching on the apprenticeship model, the reality was that members of the Iokai were required to learn in a strongly prescribed, step-by-step manner which Kishi had openly objected to for a long time. Although a loyal disciple, Kishi's work had always had a strong character of its own and, despite the close understanding between the two, had continued to develop on a different trajectory from Masunaga's. Kishi had gone as far as he could under Masunaga's tutelage and was now troubled that his teacher was not able to offer the answers he craved. The teacher himself had admonished his senior disciple over the years for his creative but disruptive influence despite appreciating his challenging presence and predicting a famous career.

Soon after his crisis came to its climax, Kishi described the experience to him, seeking guidance. Although Masunaga was sympathetic and told Kishi that he had gained *eshin*, described as the complete transformation of a person's values, it was at this point that they parted ways by mutual agreement. While there was sadness in this for both men, Kishi emerged through his trials as a master in his own right.

When this break with Masunaga came, Kishi could no longer call his work Shiatsu; this name was too strongly associated with the styles of Namikoshi and Masunaga to claim as his own. Like other masters before him, the decision to rename the art was not a break from the essence but a restatement of it from his own authority, and he called his approach *Seiki-Soho*.

Since that turbulent time, Kishi has continued to teach and practise Seiki-Soho and has spent many years in Europe gaining a large following among Shiatsu students as well as others who have studied only Seiki. In the early years, his treatments would often not involve manual touch and he gained a reputation for being obscure and eccentric. Still others loved his sometimes unusual but always powerful treatments and workshops. His approach, they found, not only suggested a new way to perform manual therapy, but also offered possibilities for developing rich, inner guidance that touched on every aspect of life yet was defined by the infinite space of personal unfolding.

Many years have now passed since the birth of Seiki-Soho. For most of that time, Kishi made a point of separating himself from his roots in Shiatsu and spoke little about his teachers. He had seen for himself the restrictions that come with organisations and celebrity and rigorously placed his personal development above the desire for acknowledgement and structure, so remaining independent and determined in the pursuit of his own *way*.

Along with an ideological preference for not establishing his own organisation, Kishi also largely eschewed the position of Masunaga's successor that is nevertheless his.

PART II

IN CONVERSATION

From the spring of 2008 to winter 2010, I met with Kishi and Kyoko Kishi to discuss this book. In those conversations, I was privileged to hear what it was like being a student, both of Namikoshi and of Masunaga, and how Kishi's own work developed into Seiki-Soho.

Kishi's English is good and, in person, he communicates well but on the page this has been tricky to reproduce. Translating his idiosyncratic and grammatically creative conversation into prose fell flat through numerous frustrating drafts. The more I heard, the less I understood and the more I understood, the harder it became to find language on the black and white of the page which would carry even a spark of the textured experience of Seiki. So, while what follows takes roughly the form of the many conversations we had, it is nonetheless a compromise between grammatical sense and verisimilitude. While falling somewhat short of our hopes and intentions, it offers a unique and privileged view of Masunaga sensei's approach to Shiatsu and points to the core of Kishi's own life's work.

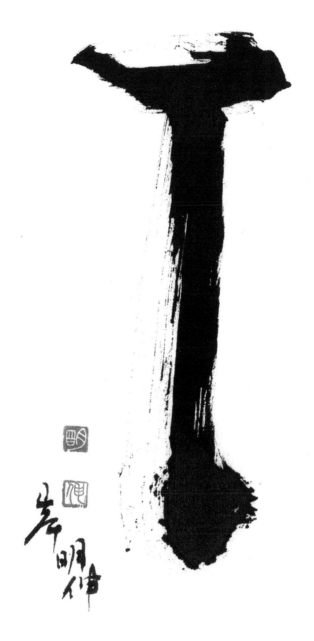

Kcho (工) Original kan-ji means 'tool':
Masunaga explained that it led to '巧', the skilful work of Shiatsu: make a hole in
the wall between two persons (practitioner and patient), by which he means *sesshin*

(Calligraphy by Kishi)

Shiatsu

Although Seiki and Shiatsu are different, they belong together. Seiki is Kishi's method and students are inspired by it with or without a background in Shiatsu. But it did not rise from a void. Reflecting on a youth he thought he had consigned to history, it emerged again into our conversation as the rich culture and intense study out of which his later work grew. In particular, Kishi was taken back to the ten years he spent as a disciple and assistant to Masunaga and he offers an unparalleled insight into this great teacher's hopes and aims.

I wanted to hear about Kishi's view on Masunaga's Shiatsu after so many years.

Masunaga's Shiatsu was great, his work was really wonderful and he had fantastic theories. There has been no one like him and it's sad that his work has not been faithfully taken up and taught anywhere. For me, I reached the end of my work in that style of Shiatsu and followed my own way, but I very much appreciate the time I spent with him.

I was curious to know what had struck him when he first met Masunaga at the Japan Shiatsu College.

He was very impressive and his work was unconventional. Everyone was in awe of him and his lectures included the theory and practice of clinical psychology, which I found very interesting. I really looked up to him and did my best to emulate him in my Shiatsu so I was very happy when he noticed me.

The Iokai sounded like a great place to study.

The atmosphere at the Iokai at the end of the 1960s was very calm and quiet, a lovely place to be. Masunaga sensei insisted that research be carried out quietly in order to find the all-important Eastern medical diagnostic system for Shiatsu. He was very strict on the principles of Shiatsu and the Iokai clearly reflected the official differences between Shiatsu and Anma. There wasn't so much theory at that time, meridians were rarely mentioned, just sesshin. He was working on theories all the time but hadn't applied them to his teaching at this point. I stayed in the treatment room for a while and they were good times. I enjoyed discussions with other disciples there.

It sounds as though his vision for the Iokai was established with great care.

Masunaga sensei was very earnest, not ambitious for himself, but sincere in his endeavour of explaining Shiatsu in a way that everyone could understand. He had high ideals and often addressed conferences of Kanpo doctors, speaking about manual medicine with a view to promoting it. For him, manual therapy was the core medical approach or king of medicine. The king of medicine was an image that came from an old Buddhist sutra or text,[53] and asserted that he must understand and address sickness in such a way that it doesn't return. Traditionally, medicine of this kind was taught one to one, or in very small numbers through experience and transmission because, to practise it properly, the heart approach is necessary: you can't learn this in large classes, it's very personal. Masunaga had the idea that it could be taught in a private institute with small classes, like tutorials, where there was a close communication between disciples and master.

---

53 Masunaga, S. with Ohashi, W. (1977) *Zen Shiatsu: How to Harmonise Yin and Yang for Better Health*, 12th edn. Tokyo and New York: Japan Publications, p.6: 'When I was reading a Buddhist sutra, the zo-agonkyo, which is practised in India, one passage was caught by my eye. It explained how the royal king of medicine should know the disease well, find its origin and cause, treat the disease, and care for and enlighten himself as to the constitution of his being. This to me is the ideal attitude toward medicine.'

Kishi himself teaches in comparatively small workshops and is generous with his time: I wondered if this was a deliberate acknowledgement of the importance of transmission and perhaps a step away from Masunaga's more distant relationship with disciples.

I was very lucky in my relationship with Masunaga. When I went to the South Korea Shiatsu Symposium with him as his assistant in the 1970s, it was just the two of us. I also had the opportunity to meet his mother and teacher and others who influenced him. He was very generous with me. In the traditional Japanese way, the master teaches like this, not in a class. Maybe you can get a sense of the heart approach in one-to-one transmission, yes. But Namikoshi and Masunaga didn't usually teach like this. They taught most people in the same way. I think that in an institution you are probably limited to doing this. But even in a school situation with large classes, the important thing is to have a sense, yourself, of what you are learning from the teacher. I'm not like a traditional Japanese teacher in this respect; I welcome questions and I want this contact with students, I appreciate it.

As I heard more about Masunaga, I wondered why he had chosen a career in Shiatsu when his academic inclinations were so strong.

Masunaga thought Acupuncture was unscientific and, to begin with, he thought this about Shiatsu too. So he tried to understand and explain it through an academic approach at first, but eventually he found himself personally drawn to it and understood its importance through his own experience. Not only this, but also his research led him to the understanding that the original core of Japanese medicine is manual therapy, based on a philosophical view of what it is to be a human being. The fact that it had been pushed almost out of view over the centuries raises questions, but it didn't change the fact, for him, and for me, that it is the most effective medicine.

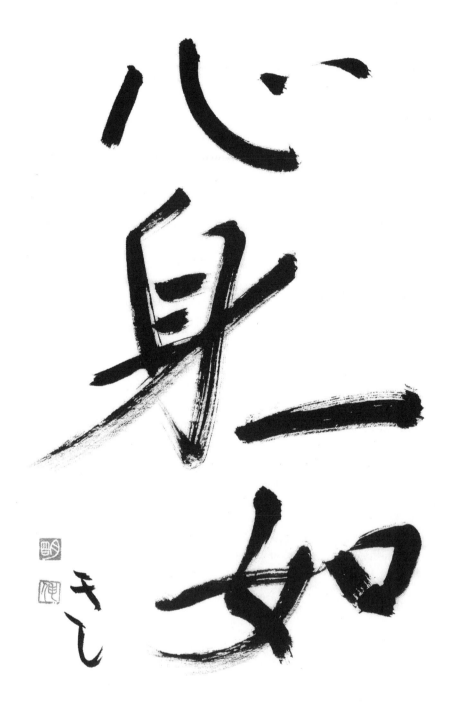

Shin-shin ichi-nyo; Mind/body is one

The Eastern account of what it is to be human is different from that in many Western philosophies.

In Eastern philosophy, life-and-death are one; both are part of nature. Mind/body is one. We have many simple examples of this as when we feel fear and the body feels cold and the face becomes pale or when we're happy, which has quite different and visible effects on the body. When the body changes, the mind changes. When the mind changes, the body changes. There is weight in the way of the body. In the West, mind and body are thought of as separate and the body doesn't usually count for much. But our hearts and minds are not separate from our bodies, they are the same. Human beings are filled with original joy. It is not truly alive that cannot be felt, this is a body thing; there's no separation.

And Masunaga's Shiatsu was a deliberate return to an Eastern philosophical approach.

In his book, *Shiatsutherapy*, Masunaga said that Anma-Doin was at the heart of Chinese medicine and Kanpo. What he wanted was for manual therapy, this time in the form of Shiatsu, to be put back at the heart of traditional medicine. Medical *treatment* that is, not medicine. Manual therapy is the starting point for all traditional practitioners, so training the hands is something you need to take very seriously. Masunaga noted that the scientific view of medicine, which is based on dissection of the dead body and analysis, had become the underlying model even in traditional medicine. He found that traditional practitioners work with this mindset, so their practice was already distorted and he was tireless in pursuing a renaissance of traditional medicine based on Eastern principles. You really can't do Shiatsu with a scientific mind; it takes you back to basics, to a more primitive connection with the patient.

Masunaga's research took him deep into the history of traditional medicine, searching for a theoretical bedrock on which he could found Shiatsu and restore it to its proper position.

Masunaga's research took him into Acupuncture theory looking for traces of manual therapy and clues to a theory for Shiatsu. In Acupuncture, manual diagnosis is called sesshin and there were two elements to it: *setsumyaku* and *sekkei*. The acupuncturist will find tsubos through setsumyaku, which is pulse diagnosis. Sekkei is no longer used much but was said to be the action of using the whole hand to stroke down the meridian for diagnosis and Masunaga believed it was the closest thing in Acupuncture theory to Shiatsu. However, as he looked further into historical Acupuncture, he found evidence to suggest that this was not the original understanding of sekkei and that the description of it as stroking was mistaken. He thought that sekkei was originally performed with stable pressure using the whole hand. This conformed very well to his idea of sesshin in Shiatsu, which uses stable pressure for syo diagnosis.[54] He was certain that he had found an important theoretical link to Shiatsu in the history of traditional medicine that could help legitimise it. As a result of this research, sesshin became his ideal way, the essence of Shiatsu, and this is what he taught at the Iokai.

Masunaga remains an unusual figure in the history of manual therapy because his academic acuity was highly developed, which the history of his research amply demonstrates.

I looked into the process of Masunaga's studies many years ago and then put it all aside. Just recently I was going through it all again and it's really very interesting. The evolution of his thought is clearly reflected in his early writing.

Kishi kept these articles and, revisiting them after all these years, made sense of them in ways he had not done first time around.

These articles were not widely published, so I'm lucky to have them. Masunaga sensei left the Japan Shiatsu College before my second year and everything relating to him there was promptly thrown away. By chance I found a thick bundle of Shiatsu Association periodicals in a rubbish bin there. Masunaga had contributed articles to every edition and they're very interesting, more so than all the books he wrote later; you can see how his mind was working and what he was researching in these papers. Then, from 1969 to 1979 I was close to him at the Iokai, so had a continuous line of contact and could see how his work developed in that period too. His progression ran like this: in 1962, he was looking at Koho Anma and Shiatsu. He put together the principles

---

54   Syo diagnosis is Eastern diagnosis.

of Koho Anma with Shiatsu, that is *kyo/jitsu hosya*[55] and Shiatsu. He was also interested in the differences between Anma and Shiatsu in line with the official research he was involved in. By 1964, he was looking at Shiatsu and pathology, the meaning of diagnosis in Shiatsu, and connecting the names of diseases with kyo/jitsu diagnosis. Then in 1964–1965 traditional Japanese medicine (Kanpo) and psychotherapy had taken his interest. He said that touch manifests people's desire for attention and influences their hearts and bodies and is thus connected with syo diagnosis. He was particularly interested in the work of Carl Rogers because his idea of unconditional positive regard seemed to be in line with Masunaga's view that the key to medicine is the presence or attitude of the practitioner. But in traditional Japanese society, psychotherapy doesn't make sense and Masunaga's use of it was seen as scandalous in the world of conventional Eastern medicine in Japan for he said that Eastern medicine is soul therapy. It's hard for Westerners to appreciate just how outrageous this was. Shiatsu and traditional therapies automatically work with the psychological, so separating mind and body makes no sense. Psychotherapy exists in Japan, of course. More so now. But we have developed other kinds of psychotherapy too, like *Naikan*[56] or Zen practice, that work on the Eastern philosophical view of the human being. But psychology was close to Masunaga's heart and it influenced his work. For instance, the fact that Freud advocated sitting behind his patients was why Masunaga would always work by first sitting behind people in *seiza*,[57] with back diagnosis. But he abandoned psychoanalytic theory quite quickly as a possible comprehensive language for Shiatsu.

In each area of research, Masunaga hoped to find an overarching theory for Shiatsu and each was an influence on his work.

By 1966 Masunaga was looking at mental health and Shiatsu after which, in 1968, appeared an article entitled 'The Recognition of Keiraku' (meridian philosophy) followed the next year by 'Reading Somon and Reisuu (Chinese Medicine) from the Viewpoint of Manual Therapy'. In the same year that he left the Japan Shiatsu College, he started looking

---

55 Kyo/jitsu hosya is the correct approach, or touch, for kyo/jitsu.

56 Naikan is concentrating on the soul and observing the true character of the self and truth in the heart. It is a self-discipline with some features of a psychotherapy.

57 Seiza is a kneeling position, Japanese style.

into Chinese medicine but I believe applying it to Shiatsu practice brought about major misunderstandings because people have simplified it and missed the point. Shiatsu is about feeling and ki and connection, it's not like *Tuina*.[58] While it's simple on the one hand, human feeling is also deep and hard to catch. You don't necessarily understand that there are points and meridians just from doing Shiatsu. Maybe you understand that there are meridians just from touch, but maybe not. The important thing is to feel first. Feeling is not Chinese medicine. This is Japanese.

A good deal of Western Shiatsu links it to Acupuncture theory, sometimes even conflating Shiatsu with acupressure, but this is not what Masunaga was doing.

Masunaga said that Acupuncture theory and charts are fine for Acupuncture and Moxibustion but not suitable for Shiatsu. If you perform whole body Shiatsu and are in roughly the right area, it's very effective while, in Acupuncture, you have to be very precise. In Acupuncture, meridians are lines that link tsubos but, even in Chinese medicine, they're not really fixed; actual clinical value is still the most important thing. In life, meridians are not fixed lines, they vary in every way. Every person and every situation is different. The sharp angles of the Acupuncture charts are not representative of human reality. Masunaga's Shiatsu chart was deliberately vague and he has been much misunderstood on this. Some Shiatsu people have criticised him for his chart because it's not precise and anatomical like the old Chinese charts, but that was exactly why he made it like that. Criticising him on this is missing the entire point of his Shiatsu.

This took us back to the origins of Shiatsu.

There's no Anpuku in Chinese medicine. The relationship between Japanese Shiatsu and Chinese medicine is thin. They're not naturally linked. When any system of folk medicine is systematised in Japan, people go back to the Chinese systems for structure, and, although it's undeniably an influence, it's not being used exactly, as many non-Japanese assume. That's understandable I suppose, but it's really not like that. The point is not whether it's in accord with Chinese medicine but

---

58 Tuina is Chinese massage therapy.

whether or not you can do syo diagnosis. Masunaga wanted to decide syo diagnosis through Shiatsu sesshin or sekkei and whole body Shiatsu to decide on the kyo/jitsu of two meridians. You could also say that sesshin is life-sympathy that touches the heart because it's about what you feel. People don't so much feel the reality of sesshin and I suspect this is why there's so much talk about kyo/jitsu and meridians; these are a substitute for actual feeling.

It's sometimes hard to wrest our minds from the idea that the meridian chart, or any map for that matter, is only a very partial attempt to represent a felt reality.

Meridians don't exist in the body like they do on the chart. Meridians are in life; they are the functions that appear when flow is stopped. The mind/body is a bit like a road; there's no problem when the traffic passes along smoothly. But, when a cliff crumbles away through heavy rain or there's an accident and everything grinds to a halt, then you see a small road that wasn't noticed or used much before. Things need to get through, so somehow this small way will be used. The small road which appears can be likened to a meridian and the factor of interruption is kyo/jitsu. Meridian Shiatsu carries the thing which people need for life through this small road. It's the function that appears when you're becoming sick. It is necessary just to see the function as a fact, even if it's not provable in Western scientific terms. Shiatsu that puts theory first is strange; there is no theory in being alive or in life itself. A child is born whether there is theory or not. Trying to understand meridians intellectually gets in the way. Masunaga said that Shiatsu is performed with the intention of understanding the meridian. You do sesshin and you feel reality.

There is an historical relationship with Kanpo and Masunaga was trying to build on it. Kishi is circumspect about the value of this endeavour.

Kanpo is intuitive medicine. You practise until you don't have to think about the points but they appear. I was close to Masunaga from the beginning to almost the end of his research at the Iokai. For me, the Chinese medicine was a phase. It was never integral to Shiatsu. This was part of his drive to develop a solid theory. It worked after a fashion, but skill and theory are the same, they should be the same. Masunaga wanted Shiatsu to be part of the academic study and practice of traditional medicine in Japan and much of his energy was bent in that direction, but I don't think that is the way to go with Shiatsu; it can stand on its own.

The academic study must be founded, firmly, on practice.

The main feature of Masunaga's work is sesshin. You forget self and practise self-and-other-as-one. Sesshin is how to be *mu-shin*;[59] how to develop appropriate touch, *tekiatsu*, and so be able to touch each person in the way that suits them best. He wrote a guide to sesshin that was published alongside the meridian chart. The guide says you need to practise sesshin. Meridians are only the practice that lets sesshin through; with stable touch, roughly along the meridian, kyo/jitsu diagnosis is correctly made and the curative effect occurs simultaneously.

Kyo and jitsu are discussed a good deal in Shiatsu today but Masunaga's understanding of it was quite different from many of these debates.

Sesshin is important because, by practising it you see kyo/jitsu, but sesshin is not *looking for* kyo/jitsu. It requires one partner to be 'open' while holding supported pressure. Then the *hibiki* or echo will be felt and kyo/jitsu will balance itself. This is not looking for kyo and jitsu separately. Masunaga used kyo/jitsu to establish life-sympathy. What's important is contacting a person's character through kyo/jitsu. Much Shiatsu these days is reduced to quite a narrow idea of kyo and jitsu that doesn't look at the whole person. It's not a theory or pathology of the character that we're interested in but the actual person seen through sesshin as something like a primitive life feeling; I don't know a better phrase to describe it, but something like primary or original life feeling perhaps. Masunaga said that Shiatsu was 'therapy of love', that's *ai no teate* in Japanese, and its practice is simple. The way into it is small, but inside it is vast. He was not only interested in effective cure in the medical sense, but something greater.

Giving Shiatsu a complex theory carried its own problems.

In the first place, Masunaga set out to explain the origins of Shiatsu and then he used the theory of Japanese medicine and tried to make

---

59 Mu-shin is no-mind or selflessness.

it fit his purpose. But there were problems: his idea of meridians, for instance, is not well understood so has been simplified into just the basic meridian chart. Also, in the West, it's assumed that you can't do Shiatsu without having knowledge first, so there is only really theory there and people don't work at Shiatsu practice as medicine. By this I mean that the fundamental skill of diagnosis is missing.

I have heard that Masunaga's treatments were wonderful. In North America, I knew of people who had met him in the 1970s who vividly recalled his touch, some 30 years on.

I know that many people said his treatments were like magic. He would go straight to the kyo point with great intent and steady hands, touching deeply, and the pain would go away. It wasn't comfortable, but it was impressive and people thought his work was amazing. He demonstrated his theory in his practice clearly yet people thought it was mysterious nonetheless. Really what he was showing was the essence of unhesitating sesshin diagnosis which was at the heart of his Shiatsu.

I wondered if Kishi had found Masunaga's treatments mysterious.

No. I was in awe of him for a long time though. I looked up to him and did my best to copy his treatments faithfully and learn everything from him and, by my second year with him, I had mastered his Shiatsu. But I worked closely with him and demonstrated for him for years, so I had a different view from other people. I came to appreciate that our talents were quite different. Mine eventually led to Seiki and a way to discern deep kyo/jitsu differently.

In Europe, sharp distinctions have been drawn between Namikoshi's and Masunaga's Shiatsu, but these lines were never so clear in Japan.

In some ways, Masunaga wasn't so far from Namikoshi in his Shiatsu practice. For Namikoshi, diagnosis and treatment were the same thing too and he felt this in every point on the body. Each point has a precise effect on an organ. I think it might be useful for European Shiatsu people to seriously study the principles again before separating it into Namikoshi and Masunaga styles, there are many schools of Shiatsu that have misunderstood the basic principles.

Masunaga's teaching of these basics at the Iokai took the form, not just of lectures and workshops, but feedback on clinical practice.

At the Iokai, we did a lot of treatments on members of the public. At the end of each one we would write on the patient's record what we thought was the most kyo and most jitsu, for instance, stomach kyo, liver jitsu, something like that. Masunaga would come round at the end to see what we had concluded. He disagreed with me every time. If I said *stomach kyo, liver jitsu*, he would say *stomach jitsu, liver kyo*. But he never criticised anyone. That wasn't the point. It wasn't the point to be right or wrong.

I wondered what the point was in that case.

The important thing was to do sesshin. Always observing, always feeling. Then you made a decision. The conclusion didn't matter, he wasn't checking that really. The looking was what was important. He was checking whether we were doing sesshin or not. It's true that maybe with lots of practice you're more often right, but that's still not really the point. The question is about concentration: are you looking? He said it makes no difference if you get the diagnosis right or wrong in the end, because sesshin itself is syo diagnosis and this is treatment. Courage is important in Shiatsu. Maybe you get it right, maybe you get it wrong, but be certain. In this way you discover syo diagnosis.

Masunaga's definition of health seemed key to understanding his approach and I asked Kishi what he thought this was.

That's a good question, but actually this question is strange too. Even asking it seems to me to be a sign of ill-health. Addressing it with the head first is at opposite poles from the Shiatsu approach. His definition of health was life-sympathy in meridian philosophy. What people really want is human contact and relationship.

I turned to my well-thumbed copy of *Zen Shiatsu*. In that translation, Masunaga says that the purpose of Shiatsu is *satori*.[60]

Yes, perhaps in a sense you can say that the purpose of Shiatsu is satori. But I think many people focus on the meridian chart because it's all too difficult to understand. The result is that they separate the mental and physical. But satori is physical; it is a recognition of the reality that humans are filled with original joy. In *kotodama*,[61] we say that *sa* means 'difference' and *tori* means 'take off' – you are *kokoro*,[62] your heart becomes one, or you could say that it becomes natural.

Masunaga was working in Shiatsu in the clear understanding that he was operating within a tradition and even returning to something more original, yet he is thought of as an innovator.

Like Namikoshi, Masunaga was following in the tradition of conventional Shiatsu. He was particularly influenced by Tenpeki Tamai and Daikoku Sadakatsu. His treatments had a more direct and physical feel than Namikoshi's but the substance of all Shiatsu, including Masunaga's work, is the art of *sya* (sya-ho) for finding and pushing jitsu (*cori*).[63] Jitsu protects the kyo so you don't tackle it directly; if the kyo is addressed, the resistance of the jitsu will simply stop. But when jitsu is very deep, finding whether it is kyo or jitsu is difficult. In order to address this, he went in the direction of meridian Shiatsu and Eastern medical theory. He put a lot of energy into understanding it, right up to the end of his life. He improved on one-point pressure style Shiatsu, which came through Tenpeki Tamai, with his yin/yang, two-hand method, a different two-hand method from that taught at the Japan Shiatsu College. He started to teach his style there and this didn't go down well with the other teachers which was why he left and concentrated on the Iokai. He taught this through sesshin and I don't believe it's stressed enough in Shiatsu training now; not in any style, Masunaga's or Namikoshi's.

---

60 Satori is enlightenment or self-realisation.
61 Kotodama is the Japanese idea that words or sounds have a particular spiritual power.
62 Kokoro is the heart.
63 Cori means stiffness.

Theory was not thought important in Shiatsu beyond basic necessity.

You have to understand that explanation wasn't considered necessary in Shiatsu, so Namikoshi didn't use kyo/jitsu diagnosis. The theory on which his Shiatsu is based is skeletal and spine adjustment and *atsuhansya* (pressure to the skin that affects the internal organs) so physiology and anatomy were considered as important as Eastern theory in the Japan Shiatsu College; no meridians or charts were used there, although of course, they taught basic Chinese medical theory. In fact, there was a tendency for Eastern medicine, such as the circulatory system, meridians and tsubos used in Koho Anma, to be made light of. Western science formed the bedrock of Shiatsu theory and, for Namikoshi, this was the way to bring it into the mainstream.

The translation from a personal talent and skill to a taught profession lost a good deal in translation and Masunaga thought that there must be a way to preserve the essence intact, even in a teaching system.

Namikoshi sensei had great concentration and his touch was very comfortable. He spoke of 'seeing' in terms of his mind being in his fingertips. He performed diagnosis and treatment in each point and said that this was the most important thing about Shiatsu, this simultaneous diagnosis and treatment. They should be performed with appropriate pressure, combined in one point; he described Shiatsu as being in the relationship between two lives. But most of his students didn't have this skill. The Shiatsu taught at the Japan Shiatsu College followed the same routine each time and, when students performed Namikoshi's one-point pressure, they did so more quickly and strongly than him, which meant that they couldn't move according to the patient's natural rhythms but did so irregularly and uncomfortably for the patient. Masunaga strove to change these things.

Masunaga worked to improve elements of conventional Shiatsu, not only by introducing theory, but also by teaching a different way of moving the body to perform a treatment. This, too, had drawbacks.

You can move more freely and with more stability using two hands and Masunaga used his whole body, including elbows and knees. It really is a fantastic approach if you can do it well, but I think that few people can master it. Using his whole body in this way he was very good at stabilising the practitioner and patient so that contact could be more easily made with kyo/jitsu and tsubos. It felt good and made sense, so naturally it was preferred by practitioners and patients and became mainstream in European Shiatsu too. It seems easy to do, but that's also the problem: the drawback is that the practitioner loses concentration and tends to focus on finding kyo and jitsu. If you're busy looking for kyo and jitsu, it's impossible to have the necessary concentration.

Having studied Shiatsu myself, I was aware of basic principles but I had picked up so many ideas over time that I was no longer sure what the original ones were.

Perpendicular pressure, holding pressure and concentration – these are the three principles of Shiatsu that were approved by the Ministry of Health and Welfare. It was agreed by the official researchers for the separate licence for Shiatsu that it was good for chronic sickness while Anma is for stimulation, so these principles represent the central tenets and are enshrined in law. Because pressing skill (*appaku-ho*) is also part of Anma and massage, it was vital to say how Shiatsu was different and Masunaga was at the heart of this research into finding proof of its difference. These principles are still taught in Namikoshi's Shiatsu because this was the only school that was originally approved by the Ministry. Masunaga disliked mixing Anma-style pressing with Shiatsu-style pressing at the Iokai. I also ask people, from time to time, if they know the difference, but this is not widely understood and people don't know.

The third principle, mental concentration, was changed by Masunaga.

Masunaga changed the third principle, concentration, to *supported pressure* and this affected everything. People don't have concentration now. Maybe he didn't mean to change it so much, but that was the result. Concentration is a focusing of mind/spirit; gathering yourself to one point. It's like a magnifying glass catching the sun and focusing all the light and heat on one point. In Shiatsu you do so with no attachment to any idea of cure. Masunaga changed it consciously but, in practice, I think that it was lost from both styles. Sesshin is the only practice of Shiatsu and it's without ego. Supported pressure and use of the elbow, in which treatment could be performed quite naturally, was a great innovation and it's sad that it gave so much stabilisation that concentration was lost. It became an 'easy' style, a way of using the body weight or 'relaxed pressure' in Masunaga-style Shiatsu. Tekiatsu with concentration is then lost and syo diagnosis can't be performed. But still, I think if sesshin is performed sincerely, there won't be a problem. That said, I haven't met many practitioners who perform syo diagnosis.

The consequences of Masunaga's change to the principles of Shiatsu were far-reaching.

Maybe it's because of this change that theory has been put ahead of practical Shiatsu. Since many people do not have this understanding of the basic, practical, principles of Shiatsu, schools have produced their own styles. That's why Masunaga Shiatsu appears in so many forms that compete with one another. People put theory first, *then* practice. This is not the Shiatsu I studied with him. Namikoshi himself used mental concentration of the whole body through thumb pressure. But most of his disciples found this hard to do.

I wanted to know what Kishi thought of supported pressure.

The sense of stability was certainly an improvement over the one-point pressure style. Though I wonder, maybe it was really only Masunaga who could do this, it was his style. Anyway, I practised it a great deal and really did my best, but even back then I felt its limits. I found an old notebook just recently and I was most surprised to find that, even back then, in the early 1970s, I was questioning supported pressure. On the other hand, I think this change is sometimes overemphasised. When people look at the changes Masunaga made, his style stands out and Namikoshi's disciples naturally say it's not correct to use the elbows and knees but I think they overdo this difference to make a point. Students now know only one style or the other, because these styles are thought to be so different, and that causes misunderstandings.

Sesshin was the core of Masunaga's work but it's not widely understood in Japan nor in the West where cultural differences have contributed to misunderstandings.

Masunaga clarified the distinction between sesshin and medical palpation and emphasised it. That is, sesshin is 'life-sympathy', which touches the heart. For the translation of his book, *Shiatsu*, into English, his work was called *Zen Shiatsu*. He called his Shiatsu 'keiraku sesshin Shiatsu' in Japan, not Zen Shiatsu. It was a marketing decision, but it suited his practice and he approved the name. In my opinion, Masunaga's Shiatsu can be called Zen Shiatsu because sesshin exists in Zen practice also; it's the same spirit.

Zen and Masunaga's Shiatsu shared a particular feeling and aim.

Masunaga had a very deep understanding of Zen. One of his professors at Kyoto University was Koji Sato, a major authority on the subject. His Shiatsu shared the Zen aim of no-mind. In Zen, a sesshin is a period of three days, usually, when people sit together in *zazen*,[64] and walk, eat, everything together. It's great but it's hard too, there's no talking but you're all together as one. So it's a different thing from Shiatsu of course, and is written differently though maybe you can use the same kanji. The similarity in sesshin doesn't refer to the sitting or to meditation but to joining together as one, the desire to be one. This is very much what Masunaga's Shiatsu was about and, in this respect, sesshin in Zen and sesshin in Shiatsu share the same purpose and feeling. His work had the same quality of concentration as Zen in requiring that you develop mu-shin or an innocent mind and become one with the patient. This mustn't be confused with meditation. Zen is action; you don't just sit with a koan and think about it, the question is what do you *feel*? It's not at all easy to become innocent. Mu-shin is about how to lose the ego and is a central part of Zen. Masunaga thought modern people could no longer understand mind/spirit concentration; even so, I don't think he meant to change this point of Shiatsu so completely.

---

64 Zazen is Zen meditation; it is a practice of just sitting.

Mu-shin is a state of no-mind, not blank that is, but *innocent* or *selfless*.

Mu-shin is like the child's mind and the goal is to achieve this state as adults, consciously. It's not a cessation of thought, it's not possible to stop thinking, but we can develop the capacity to allow our thoughts to pass through and not become stuck. Shiatsu is performed with this empty-mind rather than from theory.

Masunaga said in *Zen Shiatsu* that 'without knowledge of oriental philosophy you will not be able to comprehend the meaning of life and therefore administer Shiatsu incorrectly.'[65]

Reading Japanese philosophy is important for some people and it can help. But that's not the same as experience. You can only understand this philosophy through direct experience and for that you need to practise from the right principles. When we say that you need a view of Japanese philosophy to practise Shiatsu this means mu-shin. Just practise innocently; of course it's not so easy. Shiatsu books have become very complicated and theoretical and this is not what is meant by philosophy.

The use of the word 'diagnosis' was tricky since it became obvious that we sometimes meant different things by it and occasionally spoke at cross-purposes.

Shiatsu diagnosis is not like medical diagnosis. In medicine, the doctor names the illness but in Shiatsu you have to understand the whole person. If Shiatsu people think that diagnosis is just, '*this* is kyo and *this* is jitsu' [pointing to different parts of the body], then this is like doctors naming a disease. I can say this too, but what does it mean? My interest is in how to use kyo to balance kyo/jitsu. This is about understanding the human being – seeing the character and susceptibility of the patient. Western medicine rests on the idea of knowledge and categories of things and this is different from sesshin. The patient isn't interested in being classified, they simply want to feel better. Shiatsu doesn't analyse in a scientific way because what we are interested in are lives and you can't categorise a life. If you make contact with the whole person then their whole character

---

65   Masunaga, S. with Ohashi, W. (1977) *Zen Shiatsu: How to Harmonise Yin and Yang for Better Health*, 12th edn. Tokyo and New York: Japan Publications, p.5.

comes to you without analysis. It's dynamic and there's no judgement. It's essential to develop a good patient–practitioner relationship for therapy.

Kishi's description of Shiatsu diagnosis emphasised quality of touch or tekiatsu and syo diagnosis.

Shiatsu is therapy through life-sympathy. A person's personality and character are the differences in distortion of the mind/body. This distortion is what makes up a life. Our being alive is this distortion continuing and changing, and the phenomenon which appears in this distortion might be called kyo/jitsu. When this distortion gets fixed or set, then it becomes a pathological change and shows up as a certain kind of stiffness or knot in the body. The function that appears in this condition is a meridian which you can call the movement of kyo/jitsu. In Shiatsu, hosya is performed according to this kyo/jitsu and balances it. This is meridian Shiatsu. To do this, it's necessary to see syo. Syo is the diagnosis of Eastern medicine in which you understand what this particular life wants at this moment. In seeing that, the person's vitality comes to the surface. The treatment itself is syo diagnosis. Diagnosis and therapy are performed simultaneously; naturally, without asking. Talking is not so certain. This is unquestioning sesshin. The hand just goes to the right place. Using life-sympathy, and pulling out the vitality which the person originally has, results in cure. The path of cure displays itself. In Shiatsu, this is called tekiatsu or appropriate touch.

Syo diagnosis was, at first, something Masunaga thought you would look for, but he changed this view.

In 1978, Masunaga wrote an essay, *The Essence of Oriental Medicine,*[66] saying that syo is not seen from looking for something; this was a new direction for him. He said that syo comes, itself, to be seen. Masunaga was moving from meridian philosophy here towards *shinsen-jitsu*, the self-healing art of Eastern philosophy. Then, in 1980, just before he died, Masunaga spoke about the theory behind his work further. He said that human existence *is* the distortion. Good and bad exists only for humans. You could say that good and bad doesn't exist for god.

---

66   In Masunaga, S. (1983) *Meridians and Shiatsu.* Tokyo: Ido no Nihon-sya.

Anyway, separating good and bad is an error. This separate thinking is the beginning of the mistake. It is this separation that makes the mistake of human existence or humans make the separation.

It can be difficult for people to grasp Eastern diagnosis when the model we use, mostly unconsciously, is the scientific one.

Syo diagnosis is not a thing that's subdivided like in the science of Western medicine which acts directly on the symptoms of sickness. You see, even though Shiatsu doesn't name a disease, treatment is still possible though practical application, it is achieved through dynamic life-sympathy. Syo diagnosis through life-sympathy uses four kinds of Kanpo diagnostic skills. These are bo-shin, bun-shin, mon-shin and sesshin (setsu-shin).[67] In practice these were always combined in order to decide on the best medical approach for each patient and these aspects of diagnosis are really describing the process through which the medical practitioner understands the patient. But, according to Masunaga's original interpretation, it was sesshin that was the vital element in promoting the essential point of life-sympathy in this process of treatment as syo diagnosis. That said, it is a good relationship between doctor and patient that is the most important key to diagnosis.

Seeing a person's reality without judgement is key.

You need to see with intuitive integrated observation, the person's whole situation as a living being is appreciated this way. Masunaga believed in using kyo and jitsu to achieve this and emphasised the necessity of having life-sympathy. In aiming to understand a patient, Eastern diagnosis does not look for pathological change but sympathises with their sense of incongruity and, because the practitioner sees the patient's reality with non-judgemental sympathy, the patient becomes relaxed and open. This is why he thought it was important to touch the whole body, as basic Shiatsu practice, in order to see the whole picture. It also needs concentration.

---

67 Bo-shin, bun-shin, mon-shin and sesshin (setsu-shin) are elements of Kanpo diagnosis,
    respectively: observation, sound, questioning and touch.

Forming a theory of syo diagnosis posed problems.

Syo diagnosis is a dynamic act and practical concept; it guides treatment only according to the moment. It's always changing according to the patient's needs as these constantly alter. The practitioner masters the art of understanding the human condition through kokoro (the heart), so it's difficult. In Acupuncture and traditional Japanese medicine, it's said that you find exactly the right key to unlock a person's condition. This implies that there must be a key to find, but Masunaga said this is not the case in Shiatsu. In any case, what is this 'key' meant to be the solution to? Solving what? The person? There can never be exactly the right key. In syo diagnosis or syoshindan, diagnostics is dynamic; it's about life. The main element in Shiatsu is the palm of the hand. With pressing down and holding this pressure, a heart connection arises. If there is only one key for the whole person, then this is static diagnosis. That's OK, but it's not Shiatsu. Syo diagnosis in Shiatsu is responsive in every moment to change and touch is adjusted to follow diagnosis; this requires great attention. I think that the main thing when concentrating on syo is to be interested in the person and maintain continued observation. This is not trying to see a meridian, but rather seeing a life.

Syoshindan – is this following diagnosis?

Treatment and diagnosis are in the same moment and always changing, following kyo/jitsu. It is necessary to use the most suitable contact, and the points where your partner wants to be touched and which are naturally 'touchable'. This is *zui-syo*, the treatment of following syo in the moment.

Kishi had said that sesshin was becoming one with the patient, or fusion.

Fusion isn't just in Shiatsu, but in many kinds of therapy. Masunaga thought it was important to feel fusion with the patient and in his idea of sesshin, two people become one. He often used the idea of a 'graft' as an example. He meant being together as one. It's telepathy or human relationship, like when you're attracted to someone and there's a frisson or atmosphere which that person brings about so you approach and talk intimately. You want to get to know this person better, touch them and be one with them. Like a tree graft. Two naturally become one through applying the hands with intent. But it's hard to describe. In this way, I think there's a difference in sensibility between East and West. What I'm talking about is a heart feeling. Masunaga said you need to feel this fusion for syoshindan, but it can cause problems because there is potential for confusion and feelings can arise because you lose sight of the other person as separate. So the practitioner has to be very strong and disciplined because it's demanding.

Comfortable touch, which invigorates mind and body, is crucial.

Shiatsu touch is fusion, the fusion is fundamental to Shiatsu. Then kyo/jitsu hosya – understanding the right approach for each person. The real meaning of touch is making natural, easy, human contact. Knowing what will affect each individual is diagnosis.

In order to make Shiatsu more possible to grasp intellectually, Masunaga would separate out complexities into their constituent parts, but this inevitably reduces it.

Hosya is the touch skill for the treatment of kyo/jitsu. You choose suitable touch, tekiatsu. If you use sesshin life-sympathy, then the hand which perceives kyo/jitsu has already done hosya. If there is a feeling of both people as one, hosya is being performed simultaneously. If you use sya on a jitsu place, it's a very nice feeling, it has a feeling of something coming out. But ho is more about sickness. The image in ho is of joining missing parts together. Masunaga separated kyo and jitsu because he found it easier to explain it in this way, but it's not the reality. In Zen there is no separation but there is also separation; a paradox. It's like how to catch the wind. Very hard to make into a theory, it is receptivity. The question is how to develop receptivity. Masunaga often said that Shiatsu is deep and not easily done. It's important to take some pains to learn it and this requires self-discipline; you have to want to know.

I wanted to know what Masunaga's approach to hara diagnosis was.

He never did hara diagnosis in the way people are taught in the West. Mostly he said people's displeasure and pain in life-sympathy could be understood through hara diagnosis. He performed hara and back diagnosis and sesshin, but hara diagnosis in Europe doesn't have the skill of this sesshin and this is a deformation of Shiatsu. In the European style of touching that is like manipulation or scanning, people focus on discerning differences in texture with the hands. It is almost impossible to feel kyo/jitsu in this way. It is different from the sesshin that Masunaga used which leads to hibiki or life-sympathy and uses all the senses with the heart, or a primitive feeling through holding pressure.

What was this 'primitive life feeling' that Masunaga talked of?

Life-sympathy is about sensation; it's primitive, the feeling of a life. It's important to appreciate that the characteristic of the mind/body of each particular master is unique to that person. Their method reflects what type of person they are. You are not Namikoshi or Masunaga. The important thing is not to try and be someone else but to continue observing; continue with an attitude which aims towards understanding a partner. This is 'life-sympathy' – recognising the patient's pain. It is also recognition of a meridian. It's not copying the line of a meridian. Namikoshi called it the 'mother's mind' and Masunaga called it 'touch with love'. It's the heart so it's not fixed but always in flow.

So perhaps Shiatsu as a whole could be described as life-sympathy.

It's not so much about pressing or pushing or even tsubos or meridians, it's not stimulation either, it is tekiatsu or suitable touch. Shiatsu is life-sympathy performed with discipline to develop mu-shin. But Masunaga's revolution wasn't finished. It was never proved and it's still evolving. On his deathbed, Masunaga said that he wanted people to carry on with his meridian philosophy but there are many new views about Shiatsu. Some say it's an art, maybe it's ki culture. It is certainly not putting a theory into practice. You can't explain it in words and then do it.

I'd heard so much about how great Masunaga was: did anyone ever challenge him?

Nobody in Shiatsu said if they agreed with him or not. People just did what he told them; he was very forceful and it was hard to question him. When someone asked a question that didn't interest him, he didn't answer. When he did answer, it went over the heads of the questioner.

He explained Shiatsu in difficult terms that Shiatsu people didn't understand. Also, the medical doctors he worked with didn't understand the philosophy that was central to the work; you have to understand something to disagree with it. So Masunaga was on his own. Even with his writing, no one reacted. He was amazed; he wrote all these ideas down in books and articles and no one ever said anything. On the other hand, he spent a lot of time addressing doctors of Eastern medicine and, in that arena, when he said that manual therapy achieves a concrete expression of a person's heart and that Eastern medicine is 'soul medicine', he came up against some strong opposition. The Society of Eastern Medicine practised traditional medicine, but even they were really working within a scientific framework and didn't agree with what he said. It was they who thought his attempts to explain Shiatsu through psychology were scandalous.

I wanted to know what Masunaga's attitude to Shiatsu being exported was.

I think his medical revolution was just aimed at Japan, but I'm not sure. He was happy that I went to Paris and I enjoyed getting letters from him and other members of the Iokai, but he didn't push me to go there and he didn't seem to have any ambition to spread Shiatsu elsewhere himself, although he was pleased if his disciples did. He was as busy as he wanted to be, selecting talented people for the Iokai, which had two branches, and going to conferences. He didn't think in terms of success. He had a prescience about it spreading abroad though.

Kishi has taught in Europe for decades and most of his students are Shiatsu practitioners, but he finds that Shiatsu has not really translated itself from Japan.

Western Shiatsu is often mixed with Anma and massage. Anma is OK, but it's different from Shiatsu. Shiatsu came more from Koho Anma and Anpuku. What I think would be good is if people understood what Shiatsu is and then they can decide whether to do Anma or Shiatsu or something else. In Shiatsu, diagnosis and treatment are not separate. In this sense, I can say that there is no one doing Shiatsu treatment in the West because this is not understood. Practise until your body can naturally move automatically, without thinking. I could call this 'intuition', but this can be misunderstood; it would be great if you could do Shiatsu through intuition but intuition doesn't work without trained natural movement. If you do this sincerely this is great and I think that you will find your own way. It's important to know what you're doing. It's understandable that people don't though, because so few people are really doing Shiatsu that it's not available. If you never get the chance to experience this quality of touch, then how could you possibly know what you're aiming for? So I do understand this problem.

Can we pick up this way of working and perform it now?

I hope so. No one is teaching it. But I think that if people really want to do Shiatsu, then they must concentrate on the three principles and on sesshin. People want to go beyond Masunaga's work but you can't go beyond it without knowing it first.

Kishi seemed fond of his teacher and spoke of him with great respect.

I am very connected to the spirit of Masunaga. Looking back now at all my years in Seiki and Shiatsu I see Masunaga's work more clearly. His ideas were wonderful and I have a great deal of respect for him. The questions I understood only vaguely back then, I have now answered. But it's sad that no one is really doing his Shiatsu now.

I wanted to hear in what way Kishi had moved on from Masunaga's work.

Before I answer that, I too want to ask about the development of Shiatsu: can *you* perform Shiatsu according to your own characteristics? What I mean is that there are limits to Masunaga's Shiatsu for me. His theory is interesting but his practice didn't match up for me because I was not him. He was a big influence on me and I put everything into performing Shiatsu in the way he taught. I tried to work with his idea of sesshin, but couldn't find it enough in the way Masunaga spoke about it. My sensitivity was different from his. These things were fundamental so, once I'd gone as far as I could in trying to perform Shiatsu in his way I was exhausted and I came to my own way. My idea of resonance comes out of researching this idea.

Why did Kishi shift from 'pushing' Shiatsu to Seiki?

The meridian circulatory system has life liquidity. Masunaga said that between kyo and jitsu there is a cell membrane through which there is a flow that can be felt; it's a primitive life feeling. It was a conceptual separation of kyo and jitsu and made sense for explaining Shiatsu. Of course, there's a boundary between kyo/jitsu, the problem is how to feel the flow that runs through it. The flow is life-sympathy; how do you feel life-sympathy? You feel it through the skill of manual therapy which is sekkei or sesshin and it leads to syo diagnosis. Masunaga's sesshin is still about pushing though and I tried it but it was too passive and I couldn't trust it and lacked certainty. You see, what I have found is that, if there is resonance, ki naturally enters. You don't have to make it happen, ki arises inevitably. Mental concentration also arises naturally as a result of resonance; you don't have to force that either. Concentration does not arise through will power; this form of intentional strength is called *jiriki*. Concentration comes naturally, without force, where there is resonance. This natural way is called *tariki*, although it's quite difficult to understand because it's not *no discipline*, but it's not forced discipline. It requires conscious surrender and this isn't easy. It is a unification with the mind of the universe where I am supported by natural vitality. This is what *supported pressure* is in Seiki and I came to this way gradually. When I did so, it was not Masunaga's Shiatsu any more. I was far from Shiatsu in this, so I shifted to Seiki.

The attitude that many of us bring to Shiatsu is fundamentally different from what Kishi was talking about.

Masunaga said, 'It is you Shiatsu people who are lazy and it is you who are not wise. Therefore, you are wonderful. Since you are like this, you can touch the life of another person. Do Shiatsu with the intention that you already understand the meridian.' It is feeling, not knowledge. He said something else that really made an impression on me; he said, 'What is necessary is merely to perform Shiatsu.' Rikyu, the founder of the tea ceremony, was asked, 'What is the secret art of the tea ceremony?' and he responded, 'Just boil water, make tea and enjoy the delicious flavour.' The questioner replied, 'Well, that's so easy,' and he said, 'If you can do this, then I will become your disciple.' I understood this story immediately because I had studied tea from a young age, I saw what Masunaga was saying, just performing Shiatsu is natural, but such a simple thing as Shiatsu is difficult. He also said that, 'Shiatsu is good if it's pleasant and enhances life.' Incidentally, in his later years he practised the tea ceremony and recommended it to other people because he thought the movements of tea were the same as in Shiatsu.

I wondered if Kishi could see Shiatsu developing in the future.

The real development of Shiatsu would be that it would not be necessary. Masunaga studied numerous books and did practical research. I respect his great learning very much. I think that no one else has developed the theory so far. But on the other hand, the theory is a pity. It becomes impossible for Shiatsu, which is mu-shin or a life-sympathy at base, to move because it's so tied up and armoured with theory; it has lost its natural vitality. Masunaga's idea was that receptivity or interest should come first but he didn't really encourage it. For me, his method was along my path to Seiki. People follow the Way of Shiatsu for various reasons and the reason is often very simple. But then your interest gets confined to the system or meridians of a school. Please be more open than this. I would like people to have breadth of choice. In Shiatsu you can express your character. In this respect it is a kind of art practice. For me, Masunaga's method is finished because I understand it, it's not my style and I did not want to copy it either, so it's no longer interesting. But, I wonder if for some people, the theory is what really matters, and maybe then you don't even bother with the practice. But if you study Shiatsu, honouring the principles, it's easy to do without theory and it's interesting this way. Shiatsu practitioners often apply a meridian chart to the human body in the belief that this is Masunaga's Shiatsu, but this is not what he did. I would like people who practice at least to know the essence of Masunaga's meridian Shiatsu.

So how do people perform Shiatsu in the lineage of Masunaga?

If, at the very least, the three principles of Shiatsu are performed innocently, the natural character of the person will come out automatically. Before being able to formulate a theory of Shiatsu though, manual observation needs to be trained and the main thing is that you need life-sympathy.

Looking back now at Shiatsu after 30 years of Seiki, Kishi's appreciation and understanding has changed and matured.

Writing this book became an opportunity for me to review Shiatsu again through the eyes of Seiki. During the last 30 years, while I've been developing Seiki, Shiatsu has spread around the world and evolved into various forms. I studied Shiatsu with great appreciation during the time I consider to be the golden age of Shiatsu in Japan, in which both Namikoshi and Masunaga played active parts. The fundamental principles of the Shiatsu of that time are forgotten now, but this is an opportunity for those who practise Shiatsu to improve their practice by looking at what was not transmitted from the start or what was lost during the development of what is now known as Shiatsu. I would like to speak about my understanding of Shiatsu; the Shiatsu that I mastered. Masunaga included in his book, *The Shiatsu Treatment*,[68] an interview he did with Dr Fujii. In this he said, 'In order to study anything Eastern [he meant *Japanese* in this instance], one must grasp its basic and simple essence and start afresh. If you only imitate the advanced form, then you fail to catch the essence.' He went on to say:

> In regard to manual therapy, I think it necessary to take a look at Shiatsu as it has achieved the best clinical results with the simplest of methods, and to conduct research using modern technology. Also, what is important in this process is how to grasp the Eastern essence of indirect effect.

This was what Masunaga was trying to do. Finally he says, 'When the act is simple, there is a tendency to assume that its effectiveness will be less or the result to be just a placebo effect.' This is why he introduced meridian theory as a system of diagnosis. Contrary to his original direction of Shiatsu as the 'easiest and most effective treatment', it became very complicated as a result. This was Masunaga's way. But Shiatsu is very simple and does not require sophisticated explanation. I think that what is simple should stay simple. Dr Fujii comments at the end of the interview that 'much of what is good and truly valuable lies within easy reach for everyone. In other words, they are often found in things that you cannot charge money for.' I think that, as life cannot be captured with theory, Shiatsu in its original form was *random and absurd*.

---

68   Masunaga, S. (1970) *Shiatsu Therapy*. Tokyo: Sogen-iya.

But even without theory, the body feels what is real. We humans yearn for things that are random and absurd (*kouto-mukei* 荒唐無稽). These qualities are the base of our religions and arts and cannot be separated from us. That is why it is wonderful.

Is Kishi's own work in Masunaga's lineage?

I hope I've inherited the lineage, but my work is not same as his, of course. He wrote about seeing syo and this is what I do. But Masunaga's ideal is a medical revolution. Maybe revolution is too strong a word; at its base he believed that the practitioner and patient must have a good relationship for therapy to take place. As for me, my own style of Shiatsu expressed my personal character as it emerged together with the self-expression of others. How we can *feel* should be the *theory*. I call it Seiki-Soho and my aim is ki culture. I left the Iokai and Masunaga. But I always think the most valuable thing of my life was to meet this master.

Breathing Again:
Seiki-Soho

On 24 February 1980 Seiki-Soho came into being. While its apparent lack of formal technique has meant that some students have found it challenging or even bewildering, I have never met anybody who has come away from a workshop or session with Kishi without agreeing that something important was happening.

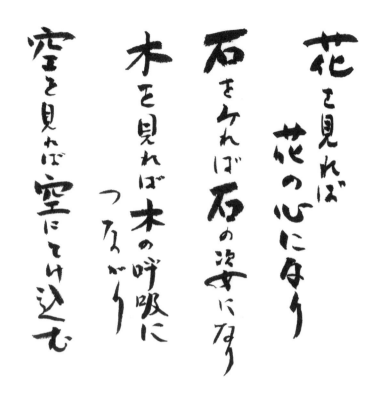

You see a flower
Your heart becomes the flower

You see a stone
You take the shape of the stone

You see a tree
Your breathing unites with the tree

You see the sky
You are absorbed into it

Anon, this poem describes the 'spirit of Seiki'
(Calligraphy by Kishi)

What is Seiki?

Seiki is looking into human nature and seeing things as they are.

> If you are not attached to things or goals,
> Beyond attachment you will be serene.
> Originally, you are full of ki
> And ki is naturally flowing and working.
> Then sickness is not necessary.

> If your body knows this through experience,
> Your actions will be founded on serenity,
> And you can observe reality.

The essence of my method is resonance. Resonance comes from the ability to observe the human being as a whole in practising not only *gyoki*, but also *wa-ki*.[69] Through resonance, you recognise the surfacing of kyo/jitsu – distortion of invisible movement. The *distortion of invisible movement* is, itself, a demand of mind/body for balance. They are corrected simultaneously with your recognition of them. This is the meaning of *ki passing*. The Seiki-Soho method consists of correcting distortions of invisible movement by observing and recognising. This is offering your presence by observing and recognising the distortion of invisible movement that is felt as resonance (ki) through the hands, which leads to simultaneous self-adjustment. As a result, the unique character of body/mind movement comes to the surface in its original configuration. This also leads to recovery and sickness is not necessary.

---

69 Wa-ki is like gyoki, breathing by hand, but gyoki is performed solo; wa-ki is performed with a partner.

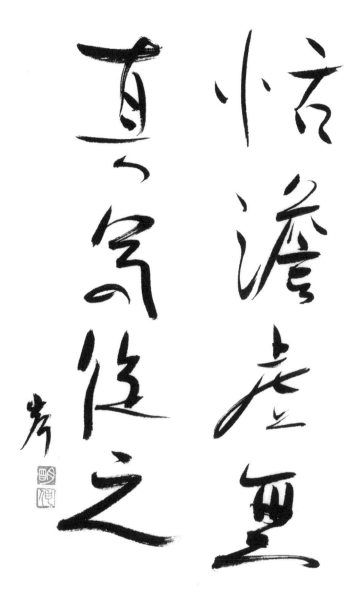

Beyond any attachment, remaining calm and selfless,
Then the ki of mind and body harmonises.

Tentan Kyomu Shin-Ki kore ni shitagau
(originally from Chinese medicine 素問 'Somon')
(Calligraphy by Kishi)

Kishi journeyed through Shiatsu to this fundamentally different approach.

This is not a journey in the realm of arriving or getting somewhere. I learned Masunaga's Shiatsu, syo diagnosis through sesshin, faithfully and practised a great deal; I tried to reach an ideal form of it. But in the process of living with and researching Shiatsu like this, I experienced dramatic changes in my mind/body. Through this experience, which came out of my background of traditional Japanese culture and spirit, Seiki emerged and manifested in the Seiki-Soho method. I wanted to come back to myself, to be free. For me this is living independently, without copying anyone else's style. I have walked in search of the way not captured by the categories of conventional Shiatsu, but which employs my character and talent most fully. This way for me is Seiki. Shiatsu was born from the form of 'pressure' and Seiki is realised through contact called 'life resonance'. Seiki is not only touching. Even if there is pressing, ki will always be met, time and space will always exist in a *when* and *where*. In 1980 I recognised resonance through my experience of katsugen. Resonance is necessary for obtaining this time and space. In resonance, both are selfless (mu-shin). They will reach the border of ki between them within a resonance space, I call this a *ki capsule*,[70] which protects the mu-shin of both parties. As ki passes between them and the kyo is recognised, jitsu will move. By the practical use of kyo in this way, *ja-ki*[71] starts to come out and the balance of kyo/jitsu is found. In the process of this, kyo/jitsu finds a balance and distortions of internal movement surface with changes of breathing. You can call this movement katsugen. Seiki-Soho is the observational ability which obtains instantaneous time and space in the moment, confirming the process of change in the living body.

What is 'Soho'?

Soho is the ability of observation in Seiki. In Seiki-Soho I am in conscious dialogue with a person's unconscious. I accept and follow the distortion of invisible movement of the patient's mind/body which always asks for harmony and, occasionally, I observe the process of mind/body in

---

70 The ki capsule is how Kishi describes the space in which practitioner and patient exist together for the duration of a Seiki session.

71 Ja-ki is the dregs of movement or sign of change.

finding harmony. Observational ability is not something I do that is one-sided, it is a relationship of confidence in which a patient becomes open and shows me.

'Distortion' can have a negative connotation, implying that something needs to be fixed, but this is not the case with Seiki.

There's no judgement with distortion, it's what being human is. Distortion is *beautiful*. It is only because of it that we are alive and our characteristics also come from this; life always moves towards harmony. Rejecting anything is the start of problems; we can accept and affirm everything, good or bad, it doesn't matter. If everyone understood this, there would be a revolution. War exists only because we reject. Reality is what matters. I correct an acquired distortion in order to brighten the original distortion that people have. Even though we are 99 per cent bad, we are 1 per cent good. My job is to bring the 1 per cent out. The bad doesn't go away but it ceases to matter if the 1 per cent comes to the front. The original character does not change but, I think, the 1 per cent, which is the clearest distortion, is utilisable. I'm not interested in sickness or health, just in shining this 1 per cent.

It is important to find your own way.

I want to say, again, that Masunaga is Masunaga and Kishi is Kishi and you are you. Each person is different and it's important to manifest yourself in your unique character. Because I came from Shiatsu, I dare to say that Shiatsu is static and Seiki is dynamic. Seiki brings out the mind/body susceptibility through resonance and clarifies desire. If desire is followed with courage and confidence, the unique character of the person will emerge more clearly and their body will become strong. Shiatsu is the performance of hosya for kyo/jitsu and prepares the whole body for *jyo-kyo ka-jitsu*, which means that the solar plexus is relaxed and *tanden*[72] strengthened. This is the nature of the human body, to make this situation. This is the keiraku Shiatsu (meridian Shiatsu) that I studied. The weak point in this approach is that it's passive and static. The body's susceptibility weakens if a stimulus is repeated. Stimulation

---

72 Tanden is the lower abdomen, much like hara. But, like hara, it is not just a physical place but a situation of mind/body feeling.

with a needle is the same. The kyo areas, especially, are given attention. As a result, the body becomes blunt instead of more healthy. In Shiatsu, touch is primarily pressing. In Seiki, by contrast, contact is with wa-ki so in practice it can range from strong and quite physical-looking contact to no physical contact at all. In resonance, you can find ki deeply in the body; this is not pressing. This is a path through ki. In this way you can reach deep into the body, like melting through. You can touch more deeply than with any kind of stimulation. Seiki is refined or small touch and a big feeling.

Seiki embraces the process of healing and does not seek to cure.

In Seiki we cherish the process of healing. If you are sick you can objectively observe your desire and feeling. It is not the direct purpose of Seiki to cure illness, but there is cure. Imagine you are a river. Ideally, the flow of water should be easy, but there can be stones damming it at points and the flow becomes choked. This is how we are when we have blocks. Shiatsu aims to remove the stones for you, so it's passive. In Seiki, the aim is to give attention to the blocks. Suggest the main points which link or influence others in the flow; the river can then flow and clear itself. You don't take the blocks away for the person. Seiki is just looking to see how the body changes or reacts through resonance. Cure is finding your natural self and talent and living your life authentically. If you, as the practitioner, become more authentic then this influences other people. They will also be able to take off their armour, which they didn't notice before. This happens through seeing clearly, without judgement.

One of the first things I ever heard Kishi say was that if someone falls down it doesn't really help to pick them up and put them on their feet. He said something along the same lines now.

You become strong and independent by standing on your own two feet. In this field, medicine makes you weaker but Seiki encourages you to stand up. Which do you think is more loving? Helping someone to stand up or making them stand up on their own? Standing on your own is stronger but we forget this and we cry out to be helped and then get angry if someone is late. Which is the most lovely?

Beauty is very important in Seiki.

Unfilled space is important in Japanese culture. This is *ma*, the *beauty of unfilled space*. Calligraphy is one example of this. There is nothing superfluous. No superfluous movement is performed. Movements in the tea ceremony and *noh* plays[73] are also like this. It is beauty. Traditional Japanese culture is unified with nature which has a background of mushin (selflessness). If it's not beautiful, then there's something wrong. Beauty and nature are always smooth or without difficulty. If it's not smooth, it's not natural; if it's not beautiful, it's not nature, it's something wrong. So, beauty is very important in Seiki. Seiki has this sensibility or feeling underlying it, which is Japanese culture. I say this because, the more precise you are, then the more economical and effective your practice will be. What is most economical and effective practice? It is that there will be no excess movement.

'Armour' is the covering that we have put on to protect ourselves, but it also hides our inherent health and becomes a problem.

As we grow up, we lose our relationship with our natural responses. We become clogged up with suppressed desires until we don't know what we want any more, thick with the armour we've put on. It's the environment we live in, the way we've been brought up, education, knowledge, delusions, fixed ideas. We internalise all these things and they become something like a thickening on us, covering over our natural movement and desire. We fill up with the stagnant energy of all the desires and movements we've suppressed. Our movement becomes distorted and we become twisted and lose our characteristics. But if we recognise this, it disappears. Maybe we put this armour on because real contact is too scary. Reality is too much for us so we protect ourselves from it. We all have our cure inside us but we cover it up; we are trained to do this. We hang onto our sicknesses for protection and cover up our vitality and natural health with layers. Seiki helps us uncover our authentic movement. It's a way of wild, life philosophy, not medicine.

---

73 Japanese classical musical drama.

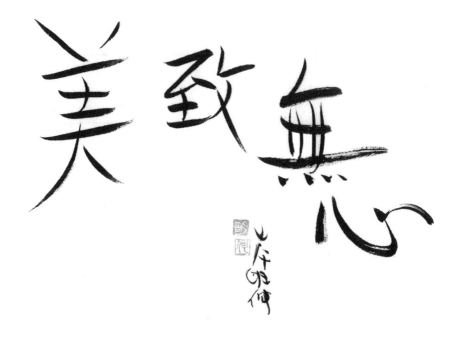

Bi-chi Mu-shin; Mu-shin leads to beauty.
If your movement is selfless, it is beauty.

(Calligraphy by Kishi)

We had spoken about Shiatsu appreciatively but one implication, it seemed to me, was that it was a thing of the past, and I wondered whether there was still value in learning it.

I have said that it's important to always practise one's characteristic and to achieve one's own style and sensitivity. There is neither Shiatsu nor Seiki in this sense. The question is, what you do with it. I always questioned everything; why push like this, why this angle? There is always a reason for doing something this way or that way. I was keen to know what the reasons were and confirm other people's conclusions for myself. If you are in a state of serene deep breathing, this is no different from investigating questions of concrete skills and selfless doing. Seiki or Shiatsu should be like the breathing when you're stroking a favourite cat. A cat approaches you with serene deep breathing. But, if you ask why, or see your Seiki/Shiatsu partner as a personality, then this changes. Why is that? Actually it is good to learn Shiatsu if it is based on these points. It is especially valuable in individualistic societies where human relations have become dry. Contact like Shiatsu is needed and people want it. I learned a lot from studying it and, of course, Seiki came out of those studies. However, I found Masunaga's life-sympathy way of performing it to be one-sided for me. Life-sympathy is generally recognised by the practitioner alone and not by the patient. It was not my own style, which was what I wanted. The result, for me, is that *resonance* could not be achieved through Shiatsu, even if I performed sesshin sincerely. Life resonance comes from ki and, in principle, both people can recognise it. When I was doing Shiatsu I thought I was doing it for the patient, to give them satisfaction, to do a good job, to give the right amount of time, value for money, etc., but it wasn't for my patient at all, it was just my ego at work. Seiki is not like this, it is performed for both the practitioner and the patient.

Resonance is the key to this relationship in Seiki and there are two people in this.

Resonance is ki, a life resonance; both people are independent but they are also together, they are as one but clearly looking at each other. It is also a return to myself. This is my style. In this circumstance, sensitivity wakes up and increases and it's very easy to make good contact with people. Both people are feeling. A big question for me when I was doing

Shiatsu was why I was so tired. My patients were happy and I often had dramatic results, but I felt more and more tight and tired. I also saw that I wasn't developing. When Seiki emerged it had a very different feeling. My patients feel different and so do I. In resonance, I do not know whether the patient is treating me or whether I am treating them. The thing that's clear, though, is that I receive the cost of the session. I say this like a joke in workshops, and although everyone laughs, it's a realisation.

Kishi talks about *looking at a life*.

The point where your partner wants to be touched is felt at the same time as being seen. I do not talk about diagnosis, but this is the syo diagnosis that I have sought. This is through *ma-ai*.[74] If the hand is placed there, then the breathing changes. The movement of the distortion is not visible and yet you can 'see' it. If ki passes, this invisible movement is evident on the body; the breathing changing and the body becomes warm. It is absolutely a physical thing. In Seiki we contact a life and a life is not visible. By 'visible' I mean, not the 'looking way' at a thing. It is selfless, it is concentration with ma-ai, and if you apply your hand, there is resonance and it becomes visible as a body reaction.

Kishi has often spoken of Seiki as 'safe hands'; for me this captures the feeling of his work beautifully.

Whatever else we may be, we do have receptivity. We feel the wind through our receptivity; the wind exists for us only because we have receptivity. So it's important to start there. Also, touching with the hand is comforting. 'Safe hands' is an ordinary feeling. No stimulation is necessary. Seiki is not only manual touching. We can't see the heart, only feel it. This is like a simple calligraphy of a pine tree. Simply seeing it, we *feel* and *hear* the wind. It is our connection to the image, or feeling of the action through our receptivity, that it touches in us, that is alive and interesting. The kokoro is in the condition of the body of serene and deep breathing; receptivity working. The question is how to come to this condition.

---

74 Ma-ai is the suitable space between people.

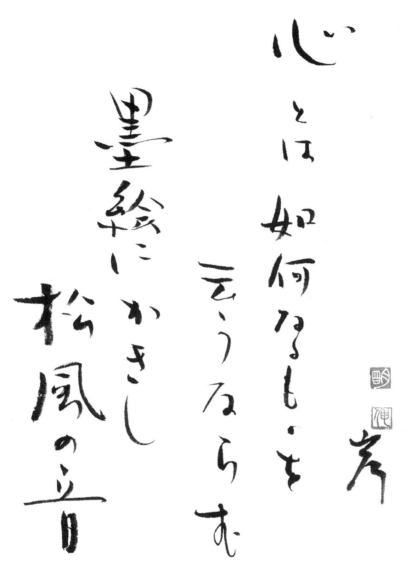

心とは如何なるものを云うならむ
墨絵にかきし松風の音

What is the kokoro?
It can feel the sound of the wind through a pine tree on the calligraphy.
It can not be visible, it can only be felt.

Poem by Betto Matsumoto
(Calligraphy by Kishi)

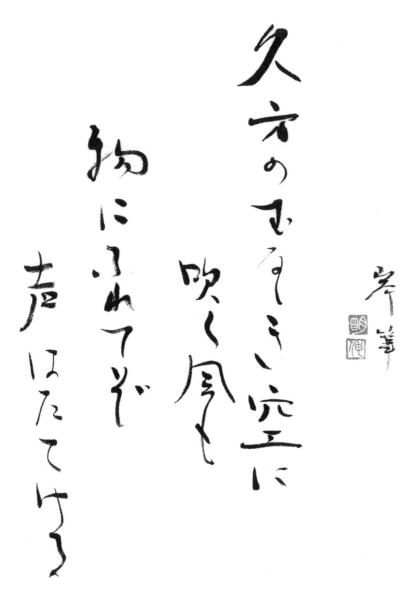

The wind blowing in the sky is felt
only as it touches something, then its voice is heard
(Touching or feeling is connected.
A life and a life want to be one.)

Poem by Meiji emperor
(Calligraphy by Kishi)

What is kokoro?

When reciting these two poems out loud, I become serene through the sound of the kotodama. This serenity is kokoro.

Kishi related a poem he wrote about 'safe hands'.

Hand
Soft and warm when touching
Spreading and reaching to every level and space
Knowing where it has to touch
No doubt, no hesitation
Soothing
Heart-centred fullness
Brings a feeling of cradling
It lets ki from heaven pass through you
Drawing out disharmony
Reborn through touch.

Attachment disappears and an easy, joyful feeling comes. This is empty mind. Thinking disappears. In this, you find your own way and become safe hands. The border disappears between people. You follow the breath but it's not necessary to breathe at the same time as the patient.

How can you have warm hands, and why are they sometimes cold?

Warm hands are simply comfortable but, when the hands are cold or damp, they make for tension. There's a feeling of warmth when there's resonance. The hands can even be not warm enough, but with resonance there's a feeling of heat because there's connection. Gyoki normally makes the hands warm, but it's best not to be attached to whether or not they are warm enough, just recognise why they are not, if that is the case. In Seiki touch, the question is not *what* it is but appreciation or life-sensitivity. That's why there is resonance. If there's resonance, all information comes to you. The question is how to develop this observation. Observation is resonance.

I have sometimes found that a connection with a partner doesn't come easily, or isn't there at all. It was reassuring that Kishi knew what I meant.

Sometimes you might feel no connection with the person, but don't force it. If it's like this then you stop. Be authentic. Authenticity is always effective and people appreciate it. What goes on in Seiki is also beyond touch. Authentic seeing changes things we may not be aware of. Too much attachment to a particular result is not good.

So, in an important sense, there's nothing to do but forget self with full attention on the other – mu-shin.

There's nothing to do. Just observe. But then what is the meaning of doing nothing? If your body knows this through experience, what you do will be based on serenity and you can observe what your partner really wants; where and when you should touch, your hand automatically knows the right angle and right way to contact. You must have great patience. This is the most important thing to understand in Seiki, but it's also the most difficult. If you know this through your own physical experience, then you will not be anxious, there will be tranquillity. This is Soho, which means observational ability. But many people don't practise enough to reach Soho.

'Ki passing' was something I wanted Kishi to expand on.

Shiatsu is about suitable pressure and Seiki is about suitable space – ma-ai. When you find the suitable space between you and your partner, exactly the right distance and angle, then there is resonance and ki passes. This comes with practice, knowing the right distance. Machines don't pass ki. In resonance, when you arrive at the border between two people, ki passes between, then the breathing changes; this is one sign.

There are classic signs of ki passing that Kishi sometimes mentions which have been put together on the basis of people's experience.

- The hands become warm and, simultaneously, the areas of the body that are being touched get warm inside.
- Areas of the body that are not directly being touched become warm or there is pain for a short time before warmth comes.

- Breathing changes, it becomes more relaxed and slower, deeper and wider.
- You may feel the space inside as relieved, calm and relaxed.
- A deep yawn comes out.
- There may be a strong sensation of something coming out of the body.
- Something (warmth or coolness) runs through the body like rippling water.
- The surface of the body becomes cool.
- You may feel a connection between parts of the body or get a feeling of being whole.
- You may feel your abdomen becoming more present and alive.
- You may have the sensation that your centre of gravity is dropping and through this your body feels more grounded or centred.
- You may feel the tension in the muscles relax or a temporary tensing of the muscles which leads to a relaxation of the muscles in any case.
- The muscles of the hands and feet twitch.
- You feel easy in the head, neck, shoulders and movement becomes smooth.
- The field of vision becomes brighter or you more easily recognise your own condition.

Everyone has a different experience when being treated with Seiki and everyone feels changes in their bodies in different ways accordingly. There are people who feel it right away, from the beginning, and there are also people who recognise changes only gradually. Even if you do not experience such feelings and sensations consciously, the internal reaction has already occurred, irrespective of one's realisation. Be free from the temptation to always want to do something with your hands. It doesn't work if you have attachment or expectation of results and look for external movement.

It is essential to seek this experience for yourself.

All begins from letting ki pass. I have listed some hints for the kind of feelings and sensations you may experience when ki passes. But you shouldn't get fixated on these things. You have this feeling only through much practice; you can experience them only through a Seiki session or by participating in a Seiki workshop. In workshops I ask people what they feel after a treatment, only in a workshop, not in private session because in workshops they are there to learn. People can always describe what they felt. They never do so with reference to meridians or theory but they can describe it clearly nonetheless. With medical touch people don't say they feel warm or light or that their breathing changes. This is quite different. How people describe the experience of Seiki really has no meaning; there's no need to analyse it, but it's important to develop ways to express the body. It's not important to know why; only that if you touch like this and there's resonance, movement, feeling, change, *this* is important. The theory isn't so important, just the reaction to ki passing. We need to change our lives. We need Seiki. Whether it's good or bad, I don't know. But we need it. I mean, there is no telling whether this is useful for present society. However, the individual needs to become independent and needs to brighten their own life. This is ki culture.

The word 'ki' is quite commonly used in the West these days and is often translated as 'energy', but this is not what Kishi means by it.

Life resonance is enacted through ki; ki is resonance, resonance is ki. It is Japanese in character. We use 'ki' in many ways in our language. You can't send ki or transmit it. We all have ki so it doesn't make sense to 'give' it in some way, we can all access it. It's not like energy, which is like sunlight or calories. People often use 'ki' to mean this. It's my feeling that energy is more material than ki. Ki culture is quiet and people have confidence in each other. This is my way.

Like Shiatsu, Seiki tends to be framed as treatment but this soon breaks down, and it can't be contained by common conceptions about pain and pain relief.

Suppose you vomited. Since the stomach had a problem, it caused you to vomit. You then take medicine in order to correct it but, since the body actually reacted appropriately by vomiting, it's OK in fact; do you see? This approach is a way of the *living* life. It is also the way of Seiki. But I think it's necessary to educate people to change habitual thinking. We all want to be free from pain. This is normal. However, the medical approach and Seiki approach view pain quite differently. In medicine, pain is bad and has to be resisted or defeated. But it doesn't make sense to see yourself as battling to get rid of pain, because it's part of you. Sickness can't be separated from health. If we take away pain, we say this is better, but pain is high energy. There's lots of energy when you're in pain, it is stress or suppression coming out. When you release this suppression, then there's lots of energy. If it doesn't come out, then this is very bad. Pain is sensitivity coming out and scattering; it is the recovery of desire, so it's not bad. But this doesn't mean that you just do nothing with your pain situation. Absolutely not. You have to know how to use it. The body wants to feel comfortable and discomfort is the body's desire to recover. Health and sickness don't really exist. There is just life and life always moves towards harmony. If you know this in your bones, through your own experience, then you will be calm and clear and can see reality.

Does seeing pain in this way render the notion of 'treatment' meaningless?

There is really no treatment because there is really no problem. We need to change our focus from what cure is or what illness is. We need to change our whole idea of health. It's not possible to combine Seiki with medical thinking. We have sickness in order to help us change and develop. Sickness shows us that the body wants to change. In reality we are all healthy but most of us don't see this. I don't say that Seiki is *treatment* because, in a session, there is no division of roles in who receives. Your inner movement tries to cure because you and I are in harmony and this movement wakes up. When we are in resonance, I feel your breathing and you feel warmth in the contact. The mechanism of our bodies arrives at natural health by letting mind (ki) pass; this is resonance.

Is there a role for conventional medicine?

Well, sometimes symptomatic treatment can further suppress the stagnation. It could be that a lot of medical help actually makes the situation worse by helping to keep the original problem covered up so that the armour becomes thicker. If you are passive and receive other people's expectations and agendas in the form of treatment, then the situation can become worse. We need to be more flexible and accept everything. Human contact is the most spontaneous form of medicine. 'Medical' means that the focus is on curing symptoms. The doctor is the expert and performs medicine on you as the patient. The patient is quite passive in this process. The medical way is looking for the name of the sickness first. In Seiki we recognise uncovering vitality and it leads to natural health.

Seiki is really a very simple approach then.

Seiki is simple. It's possible for everyone to do effectively and it's safe. This is why it's good. Nature is simple and that's why it affects people deeply. Remember that Fusai Ota said the same about Anpuku: everyone can do it. Masunaga did not like complicated Anma techniques. He researched Fusai Ota's Suiatsu and recommended Shiatsu as a home remedy. This is also why people find it hard to believe. Seiki is just meeting a person through concentrated observation. This is my syoshindan, but I don't call it diagnosis. We do need knowledge, of course, but the body is not interested in knowledge; the body wants nice feeling, life sense, resonance.

Some medics have shown interest over the years.

In my early days in Europe quite a number of doctors were interested in learning about this work. I was asked to teach medical students when I was first in Europe in the early 1970s. More recently doctors have also shown interest in Seiki, because it's obviously effective and a possible new approach for health. But they can't fit it into the medical structure they use. Even when there's cure, they can't say it is medicine, so they conclude it must be magic. But it's not magic. You only call something magic when you don't understand it.

Does Seiki use the intuition?

In Seiki-Soho, consciousness is more important, but intuition is important too because it is intuitive integrated observation. But intuition is a vague word. Maybe people mean instinct when they talk about intuition, like animals have. However, intuition does not come out of the body/mind which has natural susceptibility or trained basic movement. Do not think you need to start somewhere by using the intuition when you are beginning. You just perform basic Seiki practice: you practise gyoki which brings you serenity and deep breathing. You first bow to each other, making a respectful human relation. Then you can do *chakusyu*. That is, the first landing of the hands on the back of the person's body when they breathe out. There is a basic chakusyu place between the shoulder blades and lower back. Touch is light, with wa-ki; I say like a feather or like a butterfly settling. It means that your partner must not feel a great force of your hands. Concentrate on the gap between your partner's in-breath and out-breath. The breathing changes. This leads to resonance. If people say that 'Seiki uses the intuition', I say rather, it uses observational ability. Also, when you are serene and breathing deeply, there is mu-shin (selflessness). Mu-shin comes unbidden when you are interested and absorbed in what you are doing. This also leads to resonance. You feel resonance and can see points, then it's not intuition; it's what you actually see through intuitive integrated observation. People ask why it is that I can see. It's because I have a physical relationship with ki; that's both time (timing) and suitable distance (space). Timing is my skill for which I can wait. If you can't wait, timing does not fit and space does not work.

Like Masunaga, Kishi talks about selflessness or mu-shin; it is a central tenet and aim of Seiki.

Most important for the performance of Seiki is selflessness or no-mind. When you find no-mind then the natural order of an innocent life will appear. To be attached is just one aspect of nature's order. It's also necessary to rest the busy mind with its attachments and allow the unconscious to move your body/mind. When you do this, body/mind simply follows your desire. If you have too much attachment, sickness may come. The symptoms of sickness are a manifestation of the suffering of the mind but, if you recognise this, then your body will become sensitive. This is

Seiki. The goal is no-mind. Seiki clarifies the mind and raises the body's sensitivity to its true needs. The ultimate goal is achieving a natural flow of life which follows the body's real desires.

And, in sessions with Kishi.

The question is how to remove the wall between you and me. Then you feel the back of the head and sacrum open and connect. If the head is released, new ideas come automatically. There's a fresh, relaxed body/mind. This is connected with the lower back and neck. You need to feel this connection. It's beyond technique because it's not possible to explain. I can show technique and you can learn it, but you cannot reach the *essence* of this work. This is about following your heart. We naturally reach out and contact. In safe hands, the heart naturally rises to meet the touch. Safe hands and kokoro together bring resonance. This happens automatically, without effort. My patients trust me, but maybe I don't trust them. Someone asked me what I meant by this. What I mean is that I don't believe, but I don't doubt either.[75] I don't know any other possibility but to trust myself.

Kishi's quality of touch and certainty convey his work better than anything.

It's very important not to hesitate, but be clear and direct. You learn like this. Sometimes I make mistakes. No one recognises this, but I do. But also, it's never a mistake because, in the next moment, I recognise that it is a mistake. This is observational ability, not just for others but for myself. This is training, every time.

I ventured to ask if Seiki is a spiritual practice in any sense.

Well, what do you mean by spiritual? This question itself is far removed from satori. Whether there is Seiki or not, we already have satori. Why is it that we don't notice? The process by which we do experience and notice it can perhaps be called Seiki. But there are misunderstandings about enlightenment (satori) and I don't like to use these words. In Seiki, enlightenment means taking off your armour and returning to

---

75   See the account of a Seiki session by FA (pp.158–9) in Part IV, Meeting Kishi: Accounts of Seiki-Soho.

your ordinary nature and self, feeling at ease and free in this moment. Enlightenment is here, now, in one's own present heart. The question is, are you present now? Seiki is absolutely a physical practice because it is experience in which the life of oneself and others shine. At base, our hearts/minds are one with our bodies so there is no separation. Paradoxically, this means that it is profoundly spiritual.

Integrated, engaged observation is crucial. It's not passive but nor can it be described as trying.

Seiki is a physical practice. It's much like a martial art when you face your partner; the mind/body automatically sets itself into a physical relationship of ki. It's already too late if you are trying to see your partner's pattern or searching for something and are busy thinking. You will start wondering if you're right and what you should do next. But it's simple, just face your partner honestly. The base of this is gassyo-gyoki, wa-ki and katsugen. These are practices that clarify desire. They also lead to being serene, giving the busy mind a rest while noticing, innocently, what is happening. Concentration is engaged observation. Seiki is concentration of spirit and mind unified. This is not spiritual, but bringing all of myself to this point with strong focus. This is the practice of gassyo-gyoki and wa-ki. When you bring the mind/spirit to a focused point, then receptivity comes. Gyoki develops receptivity and sensitivity. The hands become more warm and sensitive and resonance is easier. We touch with this attitude, the attitude of 'how do you feel'. We need to look inside, feeling ourselves. There is pressing, but with wa-ki, so it's not just pressing, it is place and timing.

Gassyo-gyoki prepares the hands for Seiki.

Gassyo-gyoki unifies the heart through breathing with the hands. With gyoki we refine feeling, drop tension from the shoulders down to the hara and our sight becomes clearer. The hands and eyes are the most sensitive parts of the body and we use them most in Seiki. When we practise gassyo-gyoki we bring sensitivity through the hands, bringing feeling to the whole body and the spine becomes warm. Through practising gyoki and katsugen, it's possible to look with innocent eyes and see more clearly. There is a free, joyful feeling of breathing that comes with this.

This feeling is resonance. With this feeling you will easily know where to touch and the patient's breathing will change deeply.

Another core practice of Seiki is katsugen.

Katsugen is not a special thing but spontaneous movement that everyone can experience. It is the action of the natural body, of feeling and movement as one. For instance, it's like a yawn coming out if you're sleepy, or like an animal or a baby who sneezes naturally. If the head becomes empty, katsugen will happen to anyone, spontaneity increases, and you become sensitive and calm. If you become sensitive then a pain, emotion, etc. which you had locked up unconsciously until now, will come out, and if you recognise it this time, it will disappear naturally. This is a physical reaction and it's important because it is dangerous if heat is not felt when fire is brought close, or pain is not felt when a stone hits you. Even if you have called something a trauma because you have attachment to it, it will disappear if the desire for attention is satisfied by good contact. Resolution doesn't occur through analysis of the emotion which came out; anger, sadness, joy, these are bodily manifestations. But katsugen does not happen to a person who has a blunt body or too much consciousness. Such a person will get sick and you could say that it is necessity for this sickness to come out. *So illness is also a kind of katsugen.* You can regain your health if you can be conscious of this.

Seiki came out of Kishi's own life-changing experience of katsugen.

From my experience of katsugen I realised: mind-and-body-is-one. It wasn't an intellectual realisation. Many people are not alive with real living feeling, and I have noticed that people are insensible to this. Once I was like this too. But my experience of katsugen showed me what treatment is and my awareness as a therapist rose as a result, and I have striven in my way of Seiki. The essence of katsugen is training the sensitivity, from which you can discern what it is you truly want at this moment. Thus, the calmed heart is in resonance with the body which stirs. This is not emission of energy, dissolution of stress or mystery, it's not medicine or keep-fit either. It is not unconscious movement; consciousness is rather a motion of the awake mind/body. If it becomes clear in the body feeling, it will become clear also in the soul. In this meaning, it is completely and conversely spiritual. This is a basis of Seiki. So, katsugen is important in Seiki and I work through Seiki-Soho demonstrations which arise spontaneously, not by explaining things in words. Now in my workshops I mostly do not practise katsugen separately. I unify the precise movement of katsugen and Seiki-Soho.

Presumably, if we are authentic and sensitive, we don't need Seiki.

In a truly healthy person, katsugen happens in the normal process of life, every day; you recognise yourself. Seiki-Soho brings this process back into action if it is stuck. Sometimes the effects of Seiki are very surprising and may even seem miraculous, *myooto*. The patient gets rid of their tensions, feels more aware, more in balance with their true self, more sensitive, more human, more natural, free and independent. We give up control in order to reach self-mastership. Finally people are ready, willing and eager to take care of themselves. 'Soho' is katsugen. Based on trust, respect and patience, deep relaxation can be found in a Seiki-Soho session. This makes the person more aware of their tensions. Their mind is set free and they can let go of their self-control. When a body starts to release its tensions, spontaneous, regenerating movement might occur. This can happen on the surface or on the inside. But katsugen is really quiet and happens inside.

Kyo/jitsu was central to Masunaga's Shiatsu, but Kishi rarely mentions it in relation to Seiki and it surprised me to hear him on the topic.

Kyo/jitsu is the basis of Eastern medicine and philosophy. I studied the basics even at Namikoshi's school. In practice, I do not mention it but it exists as a background. Masunaga applied it to Shiatsu. This book started with Shiatsu, so I used kyo/jitsu to explain 'the distortion of invisible movement' in Seiki. It is important you feel how; words are not important. We utilise kyo. In Seiki, you don't try to remove jitsu, because it is protecting the kyo. If the kyo is addressed, there's no need for jitsu. If you are in resonance with your partner, their imbalance shows itself. Imbalance reveals your original character. If the imbalance clears up, there is balance, but it's not you that makes this balance. It's neither good nor bad. It is nature. You will come back to your original character or your natural health.

Kishi prefers not to give many practical directions for performing Seiki, concerned as he is that these will fix it, but there are a few principles.

The three pillars of Seiki are susceptibility, desire and ki. First, you use integrated body movement that roots the body centre. The entire body is moved as one. Also, when practising Seiki, we connect with the breath of the person, especially the end of the out-breath which is used to relax into the connection. Then, just before the new breath is taken, you release completely and give space. Finally, the use of the hand without using hand movement. The hands or thumbs are used to make contact but not to stimulate. Every moment emerges from the relaxed attention to the person. Seiki is a path of devotion, tariki, trusting that the body already knows the way.

In giving attention to your partner's breathing, their whole character becomes apparent.

The more you practise Seiki and the more you develop your sensitivity, and ki passes, the more you will be able to see and feel. It's very important to watch the person's breathing. Everything is in the breath. The person's whole life and personality are in the breath. You're feeling their breathing all the time. You follow movement and maybe encourage the distortion to go where it wants. Then easier flow comes. The energy moves more freely and the person can breathe again. Offering the present is everything; *ki-do-ma*.[76]

'Points' are something else that Kishi talks about.

During a Seiki-Soho session, the person 'in charge' will look for specific resonance points which allow movement. The looking is not so much based on seeing with the eyes but by sensitivity and careful observation, trying to find out what the person really needs. To be able to do so, you empty the mind and tune in to the energy of the person. The resonance points will allow you to really communicate with each other and triggers the self-healing process. The body releases stagnation in this process, even hidden, forgotten or suppressed tensions emerge. Deep trauma, hidden in the unconscious, can find its way back to consciousness and

---

76   Ki-do-ma is the right timing, right place and when to finish.

can be released. Sensitivity is improved. First you see and, even if you don't see, contact is possible. But first ask yourself how you feel. Talking is important too; first impressions. But it's vital not to be attached to any of these impressions. You just notice them. Then slowly these things disappear and spots or points appear and you want to contact them. You contact where there is an attraction. When you make contact, resonance grows, like ripples. The more relaxed you are, the more you contact. The hands become warm as well, and relaxed. As you do this, the movement or resonance grows. You feel movement; contraction and expansion. The breathing changes. As you recognise this, movement begins and change happens. The hand then knows which angle to make contact with and touches where necessary and in the right way. This isn't pressing, it's correct contact; heart to heart; ki to ki. Resonance. With relaxed hands comes the desire to contact.

'Following desire' was discussed a lot.

What do you *really* want? Do you understand this? Really? Unless you understand this, you won't know what Seiki is about. What's the difference between hunger and really being hungry? It's clear wanting rather than the idea of wanting. So, rather than thinking it's dinner time because that's the usual time of day, real hunger isn't a thought. You simply eat when you actually desire food. It's action, not ideas. You have to find the feeling of joy that comes when you find the thing you want. It's not easy if you've covered up your desires for many years and done what you thought you should do rather than your heart's desire. You can practise following your desire in big or small ways in daily life.

Both Seiki and Shiatsu are mastered only through body experience and are also a physical expression, but such simplicity is so often lost.

It is difficult to find language to express a physical feeling. I am looking for the words to explain my work and have read many books myself. Such research is not bad for me and I find it interesting, sometimes I find a common point with my work in a surprising field. However, even if you can devise beautiful expressions with words, they are still just words, after all. They are not the thing itself. A physical feeling cannot exist as anything other than a physical feeling. It's the same with health, you can't be healthy just by knowing the definition. A story from the Chinese Taoist, Chuang-Tzu, gives a picture of Seiki-Soho practice that I can identify with:

The Houtei Dialogue

The Bunkei King heard talk of the butcher, Houtei, who, as he worked, made a sound like music, and he wanted to see this for himself. So Houtei demonstrated his art to the Bunkei King.

As his hand touched the carcass of a cow, his shoulder leant against its body suddenly, and he straddled it. He went down on one knee and quickly, whenever the cleaver moved, it resounded with a sound like, 'bali bali'. All the sound emitted in this way suited the movements which were beautiful, like dancing, and the sound served as an accompaniment to the performance.

When he had watched this, the Bunkei King said, 'How do you achieve such a wonderful skill as this?'

Houtei put down the cleaver and answered, 'It is the Way (Do) and this exceeds skill. When I started out as a butcher, I only worked on the form of the cow which you see with your eye. I did not know in what direction I would move first or where to touch. But, after three years of doing this, I stopped seeing the body of the cow with my eyes. Now, I do not observe a cow with my eyes but with my heart (kokoro). The process of perception that is driven by the sensory organs stops and only the spirit (kokoro) works. I cut into the wide gap between flesh and bone with my cleaver, going into the large space in the joint, following the body of the cow as it naturally is. I can cut and tear where there are natural gaps. I can cut between meat and bone according to what is naturally there. With this skill my cleaver never gets stuck and there is never any difficulty.

A skilful butcher needs a new cleaver every year because meat is torn apart with it. A common butcher needs a new cleaver every month because bone is cut and snapped. But I have been using my cleaver for 19 years. It still looks as though it has only just been sharpened on the whetstone and I have butchered thousands of cows since it was sharpened. There is space in the joint of a cow but there is no thickness to the edge of a cleaver. There is certainly enough room to move the blade freely since something without thickness is put to something with space. For this reason, even having used my cleaver for so long, it still shines like it was just sharpened. Whenever the cleaver comes to a tangled point of meat and bone, I see the difficulty. In this case, I focus my heart's intent; I stop to look at the place and move my cleaver delicately and slowly. In this way a cow is so quickly butchered that it falls like dust to the ground – Bang! As I relax, I just stand there with the cleaver in my hand and look around, satisfied. Then I wipe the blood from it and put it away.'

The Bunkei King responded, 'It is wonderful, I have understood from Houtei's words how to live in the true way.'

I think that if you analyse this story with your head, it's just a fantasy that can't be understood. But it makes sense if you get to know a thing through the heart and feeling.

When people ask you how hard to press, in a way they are looking for a starting place or some structure for guidance but are not really feeling.

People like to have structure and structure has its uses, but people ask questions that demonstrate that they haven't understood so I do wonder. In workshops, for instance, Shiatsu students regularly ask me how much pressure they should apply. This is the wrong question and demonstrates a fundamental misunderstanding. Ki meets ki. This is resonance. It looks like pressing but it's not pressing. It looks like the hand that's being used but it's not the hand that makes contact. The feeling is much bigger. If you connect, you can connect with the whole body through one point, so it's not the physical hand touching. If you can find the first point then you can see the links or connections from one point to the next. You can see the dynamic of change, joined, like links in a chain. It's a ripple effect. If you recognise this process, then you are doing Seiki-Soho. If you can see the process, then change is possible. As movement starts in the body, then stagnated movement in the blocks comes to the surface with the breath. The spine gets hot as the body consumes ja-ki more efficiently. With this comes a feeling of being refreshed. This is also katsugen. The body is finding harmony naturally.

In describing Seiki sessions, Kishi mentions ja-ki and, while for his audiences this often sounds like a waste product, for him it is neutral.

Ja-ki is the dregs left over from movement. It is the right moment coming, a sign of change. Stagnant movement that has been covering up your authentic movement drops away in Seiki-Soho and in katsugen. The movement in the body results in a residue that we can call ja-ki. If you think it's bad, then it's bad. But, like excrement and urine, they are not bad, but it would be a problem not to eliminate them. Ja-ki is just what comes off the body when movement harmonises. For me it looks like smoke and this is useful because I can see what's happening, but ja-ki has no form. It manifests, but with no form. I don't care if I see it or not. I didn't try to see it and then one day I did see it. It's helpful that I can, but please don't get hung up on seeing ja-ki. Some people see; others feel in some way, or smell ja-ki. People are all different. But with Shiatsu there isn't enough space for this to happen. It's too busy. So it was a big question for me, 'How to give space?'

Something like *The Art of War*.[77]

If the body's door opens, enter quickly, like the wind. The question is how to open the door. This is like the old strategies of *The Art of War*: *come in like the wind, then quiet like the forest, influence like spreading fire, steady like the mountain.* Seiki-Soho is performed like this and then the patient changes herself, you don't change her. She chooses to change for herself.

Why do you describe Seiki as 'ki culture'?

Seiki is not only about how we can live with our full life force, it is also about how we can lead individual, satisfying and free spiritual lives by realising our full potential as human beings. This is achieved by living our life, by letting nature take its course without *intervention with the mind*. We can then reach the world beyond what is reachable with only our intellect or physical strength. I call this, *culture of ki*. When you can make a contact *naturally without any attachment or interest*, that which is impossible through just using technique, becomes possible.

---

77   *The Art of War* is a Chinese military work, probably written by Sun Tzu, in the sixth century.

其疾如風 其徐如林 侵掠如火 不動如山

Fu-Rin-Ka-Zan[79] from *The Art of War* by Sun Tzu (SunZi) 孫子

(Calligraphy by Kishi)

---

78 Fu – wind, Rin – forest, Ka – fire, Zan – mountain. It is quick like the wind, serene like a forest, attacks like a fire and is immovable like a mountain.

I was curious about the wish to write this book.

Yes, well, you can't convey Seiki skill in books. I like another story from Chuang-Tzu about this:

> One day, a King was studying philosophy at his desk. A workman, doing a job for the court, happened to pass by where he was sitting. Not thinking about whom he was addressing, the workman asked the King what he was reading. The King was surprised at being accosted like this but answered that he was reading the great philosophers. The workman responded that, surely, you can't gather the essence of anything from mere words. The King was furious. Many people wouldn't escape with their lives after such audacity but he appreciated the workman's directness nonetheless and asked him to explain what he meant. The workman said that he was a wheelwright and that, although much could be explained about his skill, the finer details could only be learned through direct, repeated experience; the precise feel of a good joint and the correct curve. 'Why would you want to read dead people's leavings?'

You can't learn essence from books. But you might recognise what you already know from a book, so they do have value. You can also see what progress you're making by reading. But real understanding comes only through practice and experience. It all starts with ki passing and how to do this, and you can begin this by asking yourself what feelings arise for you. But you can only experience this by attending a Seiki workshop or receiving a session. I could tell you about points in Seiki, the 'breathing point' or the 'resonance points'. I could draw a chart for you, but it is something like 'pie in the sky', there's no feeling with that. There are already many books like this, they're like cookery books; without feeling and sensation there is no structure or theory. The human body needs human perception. Sensory resonance is the only way to contact humans. And only humans can promote the passing of ki. I am writing this book because things are getting more complicated and people are accepting with no doubt. No one is teaching this work now, which has its basis in simplicity. This is an invitation.

PART III
MUNICH
WORKSHOP
JULY 2010

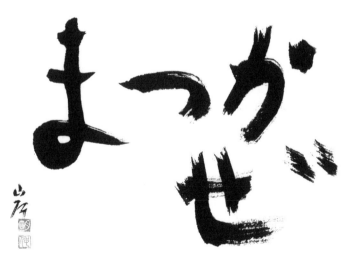

Matsu-kaze: the wind through a pine tree:
You are caught by the wind

(Calligraphy by Kishi)

Day one

A Friday morning at the end of July. The room is light and airy; windows and a balcony run down the right side and look out onto a sunny courtyard. The weather this summer has been mixed but today is warm enough for short sleeves and a gentle breeze finds its way through the open doors and windows. Martial arts style, the wooden floor is covered, wall to wall, with red rubberised mats. Shiatsu style, blankets and sheets have been spread over the top.

Twenty-one students gather in the entrance to change and gradually move into the room to find a place; some greet old friends enthusiastically, others, perhaps new to this work or the surroundings, are more diffident. Forming a rough oval, sitting on cushions, crossed-legged or kneeling, the place buzzes. At ten o'clock Kyoko comes in quietly and sits, facing the wall of windows. In a little while, Kishi enters and takes his place beside her and the room subsides to a hush. Both wear *hakama*,[79] designed and made in Japan especially for Seiki with modified, tapered legs. The dark blue trousers support the lower back with a stiff, broad band and tie at the waist for Kyoko, below the waist in the men's style for Kishi; traditional white wrap tops with narrowed sleeves for practicality complete the simple, but distinctly Japanese, look.

Kishi sits upright in seiza, eyes closed, introducing silence like the embrace of a warm bath that stretches out; it's hard to say how long.

Opening his eyes, he looks around and gestures to a tall man across the room, 'So!' Kishi indicates the workshop organiser. A familiar ritual for both of them. Kishi lived in Munich in the 1980s and has returned many times since, so he knows the city and some of these people well.

'Yes. I want to welcome Kishi and Kyoko.' He inclines his body towards them, respectful and smiling:

'They were here teaching a workshop only two weeks ago and the weather was very hot then. I had explained to people before that Seiki was like clouds moving but with blue sky underneath. But we

---

79 Mostly seen in the West in martial arts, specifically Aikido, the trousers are usually wide, looking more like a long skirt over narrow under-trousers.

only had blue sky that time. Now it seems we have many clouds so maybe it makes more sense and I can say this now. I'm very happy to welcome Kishi and Kyoko here again, it is a great privilege.'

'Thank you.' Kishi bows to the class. Everyone quickly adjusts themselves to perform versions of the bow in return. Most are used to sitting on the floor since the workshop is taking place in a Shiatsu college and the majority of participants have done some practice.

Kishi sits quietly again for some minutes. 'Before we introduce ourselves I will demonstrate my method.' He moves into the centre of the room to a carefully positioned mat. 'One person please. May I have a volunteer?' The workshop has begun.

A new student, E, comes forward immediately, fearing it might be her only chance, having been told by friends to take the opportunity as soon as she can. Kishi indicates that she should kneel in front of him. She's unsure what she should do but he bows deeply to her in seiza and she picks up the cue and follows suit.

'Now turn around please.' She does so and sits, kneeling in seiza with her back to him while he sits behind her on his feet, in an upright crouch. He places his right hand in the middle of her back and his left hand gently on her left shoulder. Immediately there is a shared 'aahhh' feeling of relaxation round the room.

'It's easier to make contact with the back first. Masunaga did this too. Back first. Not face to face, no talking, just looking.' He has a deep voice, certain, and the room is still and quiet, paying close attention. He places his hands and E relaxes, her breathing changing in deep sighs. Still sitting, she begins to move slowly, in a circular fashion, and her head drops. 'Here and here,' he says. Hands on her head, thumbs on the *occiput*,[80] he stands and follows her movement. She continues to move, slumping a little.

'Lie on your front,' and she does so. 'Her breathing has changed.' It is clearly so, her chest rose in a full inhalation and subsided into a new rhythm. He sits beside her at a right angle, a few inches apart from her. 'This is very important, this distance. The right distance to the last millimetre. Exactly right. After many years of practice I know

---

80 The occiput is the back and base of the skull, where it joins the neck in a bony ridge.

the right distance. I can feel it. Then resonance is possible. Then I can see where I want to touch and a "ki capsule" or ki shelter forms clearly.' He indicates a space from E's head to feet that envelopes both of them. He asks the class where they would touch if they were in his place. A silence ensues, then several people make suggestions, mostly pointing to about the same place on E's back. Kishi nods and looks. Then he places his hands on her back, here and there, observing all the time. 'Ja-ki is coming out,' he points to a place where he sees smoke rising. Most students do not see this but many have a sense, in observing, that there is 'something' to apprehend even if it defies the eyes and descriptive language. 'I'm looking at the whole body,' he touches E's back. 'This is the *Hirata* zone.[81] Kurakichi Hirata. I'm telling you this now but nobody in Europe knows him. He had similar ideas to Masunaga about the importance of manual therapy.'

He asks her to turn over and spends some more time on the abdomen. When he finishes he taps her on the shoulder, one hand steady, the other performing a gentle but firm pat to indicate the session is over. They bow again to finish.

Another new student, S, answers the next request for a volunteer. She tells him that she is pregnant but clearly not by many weeks. They bow to each other, he with straight back, folding from the hips, hands in front of him in a neat V. She, in the European style, with a more rounded back, head to the floor. She sits with her back to him and he observes. The feeling in the air of relaxed but focused concentration is palpable. No one moves. When S lies down, Kishi touches her back. 'Pregnant women have much tension in the arms and here.' He points to the upper back where the neck joins the body. 'It's very important to work here.' He moves his hands around her body where he sees a series of points unfold and relax, gently guiding. At the lower back he touches her spine: 'There is pressure here in pregnancy,' an area of tension can be 'seen' there.

One more treatment is for V, a student for many years. He touches her back when she lies down, then goes to her head, fingers hooked lightly round the occiput. Even with her eyes closed and no facial expression, she begins to look easier. Then he touches the top of

---

81 See note 37 on pp.38–9 for elaboration.

her head as she lies on her front, head to the side. Thumbs on top, fingers splayed to the side. 'I'm pulling up a bit, like this,' he takes his hands off and shows what he means in the air, 'tension here. Now here is relaxing,' he points to the upper back which is tight and rounded, unfolding, 'then here' the lower back. Nothing Kishi does is accidental and the class can watch V's movement, internal and external in small physical movements, together with the precision of Kishi's observation and hands. When she turns over he places his hands on V's solar plexus: '80 per cent of women are tight here.' He holds the occiput in his left hand while the right hand stays on the solar plexus.

After the treatment, Kishi sits back: 'So, what did you feel?' He looks at the people who have just received sessions and they give short accounts. All are practitioners and are touched by his work. E describes how easy and delightful it was to 'call' Kishi's hands to where she felt a need.

'Yes,' he says, 'it's very simple. No need for theory, just observation. Your body knows where to touch. It calls. I just listen.'

S says she found it interesting. 'In the last few days I had a pain here, in my back, and you touched it exactly and now it's gone. I could feel things moving inside. It felt wonderful to be touched exactly right.'

Someone asks, 'How do you know the right distance?' He answers her, 'You feel it. You know. It's practice.'

We sit for a moment. 'So, now. Would you introduce yourselves please? I would like to know what your motivation is for coming on this workshop; why you are interested in Seiki?'

Each person takes a turn, round the room. Some interesting stories emerge. Everyone has some experience of Shiatsu, although this is not the case on all Seiki workshops. A few explain how they came across Kishi and what effect his work has had on their lives. New students may have come across him through their Shiatsu teachers; one or two were intrigued by the workshop description in the college programme and came to find out more. Another small band express some dissatisfaction with the way they perform Shiatsu and are looking for inspiration. At least six are experienced Shiatsu teachers.

Finally it is the turn of Kyoko. Married to Kishi for 22 years, she did not train in Shiatsu. Kyoko's path was traditional kimono weaving to which she devoted many years, researching each specialised stage, from silk worm to hand loom. Dedicated to pursuing her own art when Kishi met her, he quickly declared that she would be his wife and, although she found his certainty amusing at the time, he was not to be put off. They make a pleasing couple. For well over a decade, Kyoko has been travelling and working closely with Kishi on most of his workshops and teaching some Seiki workshops of her own. She brings her own experience and insights to the work.

'For many years I have done Seiki workshops with Kishi. This last year,' she says, 'I've been doing a lot of work on this book. I am between Alice and Kishi, doing a lot of writing [Kyoko has had the unenviable task of translating some of Kishi's words into English and finding ways to put Seiki into words]. It's very hard to describe this manual therapy. I decided it could not be done through my head.' She pauses. 'A few days ago I cut my thumb.' She holds up her hand so everyone can see a livid cut that's just beginning to heal.

'There was blood everywhere and Kishi did gyoki on it and the cut quickly came together. I put a bandage on it and carried on writing. But, because I did that, it opened up and started bleeding again. So I thought *I must stop*. No cooking, no writing. Maybe unconsciously I didn't want to do so much writing, maybe that's why I cut my thumb. Kishi has to cook now and I relax. But Kishi did gyoki on it and I saw clearly what happened.'

She demonstrates with her own hand doing gyoki over the cut. 'It hurt a lot but closed up very quickly. This work is practical, I *see* the effect. Now…I want to show you.' She indicates her audience.

Kishi gathers himself to speak.

'Now I'm writing a book and many ideas are coming. I also come from Shiatsu and, looking at it again after all this time, can verify Shiatsu through my years of work in Seiki. Masunaga was my teacher and I have much respect for him. He taught three principles of Shiatsu. Do you know these?'

Some people round the room nod, 'One is pressing down.' He mimes perpendicular pressing with his thumb. 'Second is continuation or holding.' Again he shows this in the miming of holding a point, 'and, finally, focus or mind/spirit concentration. But people did not understand this concentration and Masunaga changed it. He said that modern people could not understand it and he changed it to the idea of supported pressing; relaxed support like many of you have been taught in training.' He makes the kanji for 'human being' with his hands, one line leaning up against another to make his point about support or leaning more visual. 'But this is a problem. Shiatsu has lost something in doing it this way. We *need* concentration.' He makes a gesture of gathering himself down to a small point with his hands: 'Like this; bringing all of myself to one point.

'So that is the theme of this workshop. *Concentration.*' In this moment he is very concentrated himself, his eyes are clear and sharp and the room gathers around him.

He pauses and the atmosphere is very still, then he asks for a volunteer so he can show his work. He performs Seiki-Soho. It is moving to be in the presence of this observation and contact where he sees points, or just observing and waiting, watching the points, although this is not visible in the ordinary sense of 'seeing'. Sometimes he talks about what he sees, the relationship between the head, back and knees, for instance. He points out where ja-ki is coming out as he performs Seiki-Soho. Kishi always works with the patient's breath; this is paramount.

'Pressing that disregards the breathing is very bad for the body. If you keep pressing, then it's just stimulation, an anaesthetic in the end. If you do this for a whole hour or more, the body becomes more insensitive. But this is what many people mean by health: that there should be no pain. But this is not health. You need to develop your sensitivity and the patient's susceptibility, not press. This is a misunderstanding.'

With one person he demonstrates the Koho Anma technique of *rikan no jutsu*.[82] It is an aspect of Anpuku-Doin whereby the joints are moved using resonance. He holds the arm and gently follows the movement of tension in the joint and it opens and unwinds itself. This is clearly not stretching but following movement in resonance. Kyoko shows the class some eighteenth-century drawings of this.

After lunch the class slips back into the room, one by one, where Kishi is already sitting quietly in seiza. He demonstrates gyoki. First gassyo-gyoki – breathing with the hands together, then apart, feeling the movement between them in a ki ball[83] then allowing the ki ball to envelop the whole body, following the movement from the central point in the lower abdomen. Kishi demonstrates while Kyoko moves around the class, adjusting people, helping them to feel, suggesting that they relax or straighten up. She reaches everyone in turn.

After gyoki, Kishi continues demonstrating, always starting with the bow. 'You can diagnose from this,' he says. Europeans typically bow with a curved back, elbows out, hands to the side and, often, with the bottom up off the heels. It is sometimes an inelegant sight compared with the Japanese. Kishi and Kyoko bow neatly, with straight backs, folding from the lower back with elbows in, hands in the shape of a V in front of the knees and the bottom fixed to the ankles. Few Europeans have enough strength in the lower back for this: 'It's tight here. You see?' He indicates the lower back in his volunteer, 'It is very important to start like this, with a bow. To recognise and show respect for each other.' He indicates himself and the volunteer. 'But it is also cutting. It draws a clear line between us.' He tells us that the bow makes the point, physically, that there are two people here and that there needs to be two people in order for proper communication and resonance to take place. Then he shows us his work, always watching the breath and following movement.

The next person comes to the centre. She sits in seiza. This time he stands up and touches two points on the top of her head. She

---

82 Rikan-Jyutsu is a therapy in which the body is helped to move where it wishes to go and, in so doing, stiffness undoes itself.

83 In performing gassyo-gyoki, people often have feelings or movement between the hands that is referred to as *ki ball*.

immediately falls to the floor and turns over, lying supine.[84] Familiar with the work from seeing treatments in other workshops, she already has an idea of what she believes is expected. Kishi works with whatever is presented to him. She looks taut, her legs carrying a lot of tension and the treatment is fairly brief.

Now, towards the end of the day, he tells the group to work with each other and practise Seiki. Everyone finds a partner, first bowing and then in seiza with gassyo-gyoki, as he has shown, before making physical contact. The room is thick with concentrated silence.

When the exercise is finished, Kishi asks if anyone has any questions. 'Yes,' says B, 'I felt that my partner had a lot of movement, there was a lot going on and she wanted to move and I could see it and it worried me. I didn't know if I was supposed to somehow control the movement. What am I meant to do?'

'It's not necessary to control it. Just observe. Allow it.' B looks pleased: 'That's a relief. I wasn't sure what I was supposed to do.'

'We need to do katsugen movement to clarify ourselves. Then, when we do Seiki, we see the other person more clearly.'

The first day draws to a close and the class bows to Kishi before breaking up.

Day two

At ten o'clock, the class is assembled again. Kishi stretches his arms in front of him, leaning forward, fingers splayed, yawning widely: 'Stretch like this and open your jaw wide. Yawns come. This is katsugen. We say in Japan that the yawn is god's breath.' He continues to stretch and yawn and the class does likewise. 'You should aim to make yourselves yawn nine times and then yawning starts to come automatically.' He demonstrates:

> 'Breathing is the fundamental condition for life. If you are tired and then yawn, you will return to the state where mind and body are natural. Breathing is god's natural providence, it doesn't only have a positive effect on our health but opens spiritual consciousness and serves as the body's expression of *kyo*.'

---

84 Supine means lying on the back, face up.

Everyone joins in; tears start to flow and noses are blown as the class continues. Kishi says, smiling, that tears are 'the mind's sweat' and blowing the nose is 'god's shit' and everyone laughs. Now he shows a side stretch, over the head, one hand holding the opposite wrist. 'Thoracic vertebra seven is automatically influenced with this stretch.' The class follows suit and the stretching and yawning continues for ten or twenty minutes followed by gassyo-gyoki as the atmosphere in the group becomes clearer and more relaxed, everyone breathing more deeply and with greater ease.

'May I have a volunteer?' The morning continues with Kishi demonstrating treatments. H, an experienced student and Shiatsu teacher, volunteers and Kishi shows the class Anpuku work on the hara. Afterwards, she says that when he touched her abdomen she rapidly recognised many places throughout her body where she felt a problem, 'Like this, pah, pah, pah, pah, pah!' She quickly points to different areas to demonstrate the succession of feelings.

A new student comes to the front and he works on her back in particular. 'Women's brains are here,' he says, indicating the sacrum, 'and they have much better faculties than men. This is just decoration,' pointing to her head, 'very nice decoration, but still…' He smiles. When she gets up, her face is quite different, she's shining, beautiful.

He emphasises that sesshin is the most important thing for Masunaga's Shiatsu. A few confused looks follow this statement. 'Is that the same as setsu-shin?' someone asks.

'Yes, you say *setsu-shin*, but we say *sesshin*, it's the same thing. But what is sesshin? No one is doing this. It's very important; basic Masunaga Shiatsu and the essence of his work. You must do this first. Before you learn any theory, sesshin is always first. Then maybe you can look at theory and the meridian chart. Now European Shiatsu rejects Japanese Shiatsu. Sesshin is not about thinking, just practise and feel.'

He continues to demonstrate.

Another new student volunteers; no one wants to miss the chance for a treatment. She is very open and the treatment is lovely. He observes her with rapt, but relaxed, attention and her hands begin to flutter, her breathing gets hot, and everyone can hear it, as ja-ki comes out and kyo/jitsu floats to the surface. Her whole body opens up. Her katsugen movement and deep breathing can clearly be seen, first here, then there, her characteristics emerging. Kishi makes contact with infinite precision and perfect timing, guiding. Her fingers dance and sometimes her legs too in an outward sign of inner change. Katsugen and treatment are joined here in Seiki-Soho, in an expression or body reaction through spontaneous movement. It looks as though she would happily continue, but Kishi ends the treatment and she gets up, looking dazed and happy. When she goes back to her place, she sits against the wall with a thump and laughs. 'It's still going on,' she says as she takes great, deep breaths. She looks dishevelled and reborn.

In the tea break someone asks Kishi what he means when he says he sees ja-ki. 'I see smoke, like from incense. But this is not important. Everyone is different. Some people smell ja-ki or feel it. Our susceptibility is different. You develop your own way. There are many ways to recognise ja-ki.'

After lunch, Kyoko demonstrates Seiki. The man, A, has been working with Kishi for a few years now and is a Kendo[85] teacher and a quick learner. During the previous day's introductions, he told the class that as soon as he met Kishi, he committed to trying to practise in this style. He now has a busy practice in Switzerland. He is familiar with the ritual, bows briskly and, still in seiza and clearly in Kyoko's ki capsule, movement starts that everyone can see. She gives space and when she sees the right moment, asks A to lie down and immediately places her hands on his back. A's breathing changes and he stretches and moves while Kyoko observes the development of the movement, inside and out, sometimes making contact with her hands, sometimes blowing. The movement finds resolution and Kyoko observes, never breaking the connection. From behind her, Kishi points to the movement happening, 'You can do this yourself,' meaning self-adjustment. He shows some simple exercises to do lying down. Kyoko continues with the treatment, looking and touching and blowing.

When she finishes, Kishi asks for two volunteers and tells one person to lie down while the other performs Seiki. Kishi and Kyoko observe. The patient volunteer seems quite stiff in his back and

---

85   Kendo is a Japanese traditional martial art.

everyone watches as he opens a little until the person performing the treatment asks him to lie on his front. He does so with a jack-knife, a slide and then a crash – the room explodes in laughter. The practitioner seems very comfortable and her patient clearly shows points, helping her. Some people are clearer than others, but then she says to Kishi that she cannot see the ki capsule. 'It doesn't matter. Just feel, don't try to look for a particular thing.' She asks him to turn over again and she places her hand on his abdomen. His chest looks stiff but she finishes the treatment, although it doesn't feel complete. She sits back in the circle and Kishi says, 'You could have put one hand on the hara and one underneath, like this.' He shows the hand position in the air. 'Yes,' says P, 'that's exactly what I wanted to do but I thought you said to stop.' She laughs, 'I didn't understand.'

Another pair come to the centre. It does not look as comfortable as the first demonstration and the practitioner looks nervous; later that day he explains to Kishi that he thought his partner looked very delicate and, of all his classmates, this was the one person he did not want to work with. Kishi is amused, 'So she immediately came to you. Attraction. Very good.' He laughs.

She volunteered yesterday and today she does the same; falling quickly from seiza onto her back, lying stiffly. Her colleague looks comfortable at first, but then uneasy as he moves to her head. The feeling of contact dissipates and he later agrees with Kyoko that he started thinking about what he was *meant* to do and this was the cause of the break. Kishi watches for a while and then joins him at the head. 'Like this,' he shows, 'now ja-ki is coming out.' And he points to areas on her front. The woman moves and gradually her legs lift with great tension, shaking, her hands rise up, clawed, and her head is off the ground. Kishi observes, his attention a feeling of gentle interest and acceptance, 'the movement outside is not important. What matters is inside, the breathing; the question is: how to change deeply? Ja-ki is coming out.' In a few minutes the movement comes to an end naturally and the session is over. It feels complete. Kishi asks the people who have been participating what they felt.

The last woman speaks: 'It was very powerful.' She clearly feels touched and cries as she speaks. 'I have this old problem,' pointing to her right hip and leg, 'and I've tried many treatments and nothing has ever helped. But now I think it's gone. Thank you.'

'You did it yourself.' Kishi tells her. She nods. 'Everybody can do this themselves. Cure yourself.'

After lunch Kishi talks a little about the history of Shiatsu, and he asks me to explain how Chinese medicine is not the same in Japan as it is in China or elsewhere; that Masunaga researched it through the filter of traditional Japanese medicine which gave its own character to it. So there has been a misunderstanding and people think that Chinese medicine is part of Shiatsu, which is not correct. Shiatsu comes out of Koho Anma, but Koho Anma was rendered mostly impotent by the removal of Anpuku, hara work.

Kishi takes over.

'Koho Anma and Anma had meridians and Masunaga put Shiatsu and Koho Anma together. He put Acupuncture theory and Moxibustion theory (Kanpo) with Shiatsu to create its own theory so that it could be equal to the other methods in the way that Koho Anma had been. This was based on Japanese philosophy and classical syo diagnosis. The most important and original idea that he developed was sesshin. Shiatsu already existed, but he wanted to explain it and include it in traditional Japanese medicine (Kanpo) which has diagnosis. Shiatsu rejected Seitai, even though they both belonged to the association of manual therapy, because they wanted to change the legislation and legitimise it. Shiatsu took Anpuku from Koho Anma and threw out Seitai. I now take Seitai back. Seiki was influenced by Masunaga's Shiatsu and Noguchi's Seitai.

From early on, Masunaga said that all manual therapies should join together under one licence and be taught at university level. Everyone should work together. Masunaga said this many years ago and I say this now. His wish was for a whole movement. If there is a manual therapy association we wouldn't need separate names like "Seiki" or "Shiatsu". We can share and agree on the best ways to do things. People can choose for themselves. Now European Shiatsu has become very narrow. As I said before, they have thrown out Japanese Shiatsu. That is why some people say I am the *Last Shiatsu Samurai*.'

Someone asks what Seitai is.

'I mean Noguchi's Seitai. One man's Seitai. He is the most important figure for "ki culture" in Japan. But Seitai existed before him as well. One aspect of Seitai was Judo-Kappo or movement therapy. This is now called *Sekkotsu* and is more like medical treatment than Shiatsu. Anpuku, hara work, was not just in Koho Anma; it was very important in all traditional Japanese medicine. Even in the tenth or eleventh centuries, hara work was important. This is Japanese medicine, not Chinese medicine. *Hara* is specifically Japanese.'

Some students look surprised.

A question is asked, 'Is Sotai related to Seitai?'[86] Kishi responds, 'Sotai is related to Seitai and to Seitai-Jutsu but not Noguchi's Seitai.'

Many people make notes as Kishi talks; he doesn't often share this kind of information.

'It's very difficult to clarify yourself but if you do this then you see more clearly. Katsugen is for clarifying yourself. You develop your receptivity and true desire becomes clear. When you do Seiki-Soho, you put everything aside. All ideas. It takes many years of training to do this.' He asks for another volunteer and emphasises, again, the importance of finding the right distance for resonance and the ki capsule.

When he comes to the abdomen, he says, 'Most pressure in treating the hara is from the centre outwards.' He shows the movement of his hands spreading out from the centre of the abdomen to the sides. 'Also, here, by the pubic bone, sometimes there is a gritty or greasy feeling. If you do wa-ki here then skin problems clear up. I don't know why, but it's very effective. You can do very well and make lots of money by doing this.' He laughs, 'Beauty treatment. Actually I am serious; we mustn't dismiss beauty treatment. Why not do this?' He points out the tightness of the legs and ankles: 'If it's tight here, it means there is tension in the lower back and the head.'

After a break, Kishi talks about the need for concentration and asks everyone to stand and put one hand over the opposite wrist and concentrate on that point, 'Like the feeling of going to the toilet. Concentration and empty mind. Very important for Seiki work and Shiatsu. Do this and have a toilet concentration mind. Be conscious

---

86   Some people practise Sotai in Europe. It is a method of physical adjustment.

of the attitudes that have been unconsciously accumulated.' Everyone stands like this, one hand in a light fist, the other wrapped around that wrist, standing firm. Kishi goes around the class testing the strength of concentration by quickly pressing down on people's hands, unannounced. Some people's grip gives way, others' hold. He instructs the class to practise this together and people experiment with holding firm while their partner tries to surprise them by putting sudden pressure on the joined hands. There is gradual understanding about the need for concentration on one point, or gathering, and the strength that bringing the spirit/mind to one point gives.

This is followed by gyoki practice again and *gyoki-hachiriki*,[87] which comes from *Waraku*.[88]

The class practises together and today is joined by the son of one of the students, O, a young boy of nine. While everyone is practising Seiki, Kishi asks the boy to work on him. At the end of the day, when Kishi asks if there are any questions, he asks O what his experience was. 'Well,' he pauses and thinks about it for a long time, 'I noticed your breathing.' Kishi is pleased, 'It's easier for children. No thinking. They just do it. Very natural and spontaneous.'

Day three

'Which way is East?' Kishi asks. There is some discussion and he gets up and moves over to face East at the front of the class. 'Hands like this.' He indicates one palm on top of the other and everyone copies. Bowing to the East, the class joins him. Then, hands together, he claps five times, hands meeting with right fingers to left palm, Shinto-priest-style, producing a loud, sharp *snap!* The class joins him and remains still as Kishi intones norito. It is a spine-tinglingly foreign sound. A rich seam of old Japan opens into the morning dust and bustle of a Bavarian weekend. The resonant power of Kishi's voice straightens spines and focuses minds. A few seasoned students join in with the parts they recognise.

---

87   Hachiriki is derived from Waraku practice developed by Maeda sensei from martial arts.
88   Waraku is a martial style of movement with kotodama developed by Maeda sensei, former Karate champion, now attached to the Oomoto Shinto sect which was the home of the father of Aikido, Ueshiba.

Bowing again, backs of the hands on the floor, the class joins him in clapping again, five times. Then he takes his place, facing the windows, and the day begins with yawning and stretching. More extensive than the day before, Kishi shows the *penguin* exercise, drawing the shoulder blades together by stretching the straight arms backwards, bent at right angles, in small 'flapping movments'. 'Children find this easy.' He points to the young boy, O, whose pliable tendons easily allow his hands to bend back while many students grimace as they gingerly press their palms down. 'Old people can do it like this.' Kishi laughs and shows the same stretch with the hands on the floor which is not so challenging. 'This is very important for women. If the wrists are tight and thick, it's no good. Uterus problems.' Everyone continues and he shows more wrist stretches, much like Aikido warm-ups.[89] 'Yawning is very important. I did three days of yawning and everything changed for me.' The class is then led in gassyo-gyoki, first with the hands apart then hands together in prayer or gassyo position. This is followed by movement of the whole body and gyoki-hachiriki. It is vital preparation for Seiki.

Someone asks about energy.

'Ki is not energy. Energy medicine doesn't make sense. Ki *culture* is important. Energy is more visible. You can give it. But ki has nothing – there is nothing to give. Energy is a Chinese idea, not Japanese, giving energy. In Japan we say that we always have ki. It's always in us and around us. Ki is here, you can't *give* ki. Concentration is most important. You do sesshin and the echo comes to you. You feel life-sympathy. In sesshin we use *sekkei* touch. You know this?'

Everyone looks blank.

'You don't know? Sekkei is sesshin. Using the whole hand, feeling all meridians in the whole hand at once. Whole body diagnosis uses sekkei touch. Not just one or two meridians. This is not diagnosis. It's not that one meridian is kyo and one jitsu. It's about using kyo. Kyo is not just here or here [he points] kyo is hidden movement or distortion.'

---

89   Aikido warm-up exercises regularly involve tendon stretches, particularly of the wrists.

He points to his arm and mimes point-by-point Shiatsu down a meridian:

'This is not diagnosis. In the Iokai the main training was sesshin. This is what Masunaga said. Not meridians at first. There was a very special atmosphere. Very calm and beautiful. Everyone quietly doing sesshin. This was the training. Very important; just finding life-sympathy with people.

There are three principles of Shiatsu, Masunaga was very clear on these points, but nobody is teaching this clearly. I'll repeat them, first is straight pressing, second is holding, third is concentration. Masunaga changed this to supported pressure. Now I teach concentration again. It's not possible to do Shiatsu without it. But he changed it and he was using elbows and knees because it's easier. It stabilises the body and it's suitable for foreigners to do who don't have a strong *koshi* [lower back/sacral area].'

He asks his interpreter, M, to lie down for him to show the class. 'Not just using elbows on the back, but the neck too.' He tells her to lie on her side and shows the use of elbows on her arm and neck: 'This is the most professional, the side position.' Then he turns her on her front. 'Here,' indicating the lower back, 'it's possible to use the elbow.' He leans his right elbow into M's back, feeling with the left hand, and her breathing changes, 'but this is too easy, you lose concentration like this.' He performs a pantomime of falling asleep in this position, resting on M with his head in his hand. People laugh, but many also recognise the tendency. Everyone can see that he uses his elbows skilfully too. He can see the relationship with lumbar vertebra four and gives it support in classic Masunaga-style Shiatsu. The changes are deep, M looks happy and her breathing changes, but when Kishi sits up he says, 'This is possible to do but, for me, it's not so good. It's lazy. It's hard to see clearly and my concentration goes. I'm not so alert. My *job* is to see what's going on. It's not my job to do it this way.'

'So, you understand the principles of Shiatsu? What are they? Please tell me.' A few moments of silence greet this request.

Someone, an experienced Shiatsu teacher himself, bravely offers, 'Shall I tell you?' Everyone laughs. 'There are five principles of Shiatsu.

First is, *don't press, just be.* Second is *two hands*, third is *perpendicular pressure*, fourth is *be natural* and fifth is *continuity*, like keep moving, be fluid. And also respect and awareness. This is basic.'

Kyoko now says, 'We were in Linz a few weeks ago and Kishi asked the same question. Most people were trained in Shiatsu and nobody could agree on the answer. Someone said that the principles of Shiatsu were to have an open heart, to work from your hara, concentration of the spirit, breathing and relaxing.'

Kishi says, 'I also come from Shiatsu. I also used to use knees and elbows. That's why I understand your problems. But why did I leave?'

An old student says, 'It was interesting that when you were showing Shiatsu work with your elbow just now, and you said that you suddenly lost your concentration, I recognised this and I do it myself. Sometimes it's possible to lose concentration in Shiatsu, like you're not there.'

E, another Shiatsu teacher, makes her own observation:

'When Kishi is working, I find that he's always present with the breathing and he makes very small movements and so he also keeps a certain tension. And when I saw him work with two elbows I thought, "Oh!" There was a completely different sense of breathing and he's lost the tension. I think it's difficult for us to practise this kind of concentration which is *usual* in the Japanese tradition. So we try to find a solution by working with our alignment and our hara and also relaxing.'

Kishi invites her to show him her style of Shiatsu and he lies down for her. E says, 'This is level one Shiatsu that I'm showing you, this is what we teach first, just touching.' She leans on Kishi's back and moves down his legs and to the other side, rhythmically, 'We teach that the hands and hara are joined so we work from the hara like this.' He says, 'That's very nice, the way you do that, but now just stay still and hold. Not so much moving.' She pauses and then continues to move around and Kishi says it feels good. One of her colleagues comments, 'You have to understand that E is only showing what we teach at first level. After that we give them many more tools for diagnosis.' E suddenly looks nervous, 'But I think maybe you find this Shiatsu boring.' Kishi looks up, 'Why boring? Why do you say that?'

He's interested to know why she might consider doing something that she or the patient might find *boring*. Then Kyoko, who has been watching closely, lights up, 'Now I understand,' she says, 'we mean a completely different thing when we talk about hara.' They have been discussing this a great deal of late and are keen to understand what different people mean when they use Japanese terms.

Everyone goes back to their places and Kishi looks thoughtful. One of the other teachers says, 'I know we mean different things by hara. Hara is a cultural concept in Japan.' Kishi thinks about this, 'It's not a cultural concept. It's feeling. Hara is a feeling. It's not just here.' He points to his abdomen. Kyoko asks this teacher to come to the centre and stand. She asks him to do gassyo-gyoki and she encourages him to move from his centre. It is not necessary to close the eyes in gassyo-gyoki, but many people do so automatically, as he does. His movements look fluid and integrated. 'How does this feel?' She asks him. 'It's a bigger feeling, my hands and hara feel like one.' Kyoko nods, she's interested in finding ways to help people feel this hara feeling and it is not easy.

Kishi asks for another volunteer and he works with Z, a new student, then asks her to perform Seiki on another volunteer. He sets her up carefully, sitting facing her fellow student who lies down. At first she sits rigidly with her arms straight, so Kishi touches her back and hands; she relaxes and the space around her and her partner opens up and expands. As she relaxes, she touches with an innocence. 'So, I make a Kishi clone.' He says, 'How does it feel to be Kishi?' When this is finished, he asks what both parties felt. The 'patient' is quick to answer, 'At first I didn't like the touch, it was hard and I wanted her to stop. But then she relaxed and it was a very nice feeling.' The 'clone' isn't sure about what happened but says she did feel a difference.

After lunch Kishi asks for another volunteer and P presents himself. Lying supine, Kishi points to his neck and clavicle, 'Touch here and this opens.' He points to the solar plexus. 'Just observe. Make contact. With the out-breath, go in more deeply, then release and there's change. So where now?' P breathes deeply, many times, and yawns. 'It doesn't matter if it's first level or second level. For me it's the same. It's more simple. Just *where* and *when!*'

P continues to breathe in great, releasing sighs and yawns, filling his chest. Kishi moves to make contact with his arms like wings, 'Like an angel coming to you.' Someone asks, 'Are you together in the ki space?' 'Yes, yes.' And there is a clear connection with P, '*This* is diagnosis and treatment at the same time (you can recognise it with the breath changing at a deep level). You know what I mean by *angel*? In Seiki, touching is like an angel making contact with you. Like an angel coming.' He pauses and smiles, 'Or maybe mosquito is the same. Anyway, there's no forcing of movement.' P's breathing is deeper and deeper. 'I could force this, but there's no reason, it's not necessary to force it to happen. Ja-ki is coming out by itself.' At the end, P gets up and bows to Kishi who then sits back in his place. 'When there is resonance,' he says, 'who is treating? Me or my partner? Maybe my partner is treating me. But one thing is always clear: he pays me.' Everyone laughs, and Kishi too, but he is serious: 'This is an important point to be clear about. Now you work together.' Everyone pairs off.

After a break, C comes to the front. She has been nervous of coming forward, but this could be her last chance. Kishi asks her to raise her arms over her head with her hands together. As she does so, everyone can see a tightness in her mid-back.

She lies down and he observes and makes contact, 'Always concentrate on movement/breathing. People concentrate only on doing: *this is jitsu or this is kyo*. Don't do it like this, just watch the breath and concentrate. Is this person alive or not?' He makes steady contact with her back, 'She is more relaxed now because this place has released and the breathing has changed. This is Japanese folk medicine.' He observes her, 'This movement is not an accident, there's a reason for it. Change comes. So now release here is also starting. This is warm here, releasing, a nice feeling.' He demonstrates standing over her with thumbs in her lower back, 'Japanese style. You can do this,' resting his elbows on the insides of his bent knees he makes steady contact, moving with her breath. 'You can also do it like this.' He sits beside her and demonstrates an alternative position, using his thumbs and the heels of his hands, 'Not pressing, just contact through gyoki.' He asks her to turn over.

'Not pressing, just holding. You can do it like this, with gyoki.' Then he lifts her right forearm and the class can see that it stays raised even when Kishi lets go. 'There's tension here, that's why it's not coming out. She is unconsciously holding on. I think she uses her hands a lot. Relaxing is very difficult. There is a relationship here to the second vertebra.' He moves to C's abdomen:

'In the small intestine area, you can do gyoki. If it's tight here, then it's difficult for ja-ki to come out. Every movement is for a reason, unconsciously. But it's OK. Because there *is* movement. She has trouble sleeping. If you wake up in the morning lying on your back, straight, then it's nice, but if you wake with hands behind your head and legs crossed, it's not so nice. So do this; release and change comes.'

Kishi is at her feet. He now picks up C's left foot. 'If women have cold feet, then this point, between the third and fourth bone, where they go narrow, you open here and it quickly warms up. Just like this, open and wa-ki. The knees and the fifth lumbar vertebra are related. Now sit up.' C sits up in seiza and raises her hands over her head as she did at the start. It's much easier now. Kishi points to the fifth lumbar vertebra: 'All gravity comes to this point. If it doesn't, then it comes to here.' He points to the knees: 'And there will be pain. But how do you touch here? The fifth lumbar vertebra is very difficult to contact because it's deep in the sacrum.'

Now he asks for someone to lie down and C works on him. Kishi says that the fifth lumbar vertebra could be the theme of an entire five-day workshop:

'It doesn't only affect the knees but also Alzheimer's. In Japan, naval officers were always very upright and there was no Alzheimer's, but when they retired and relaxed their posture, then some of them got Alzheimer's. Now it's possible for anyone to get Alzheimer's at 40 or 50 years old because there's no flexibility here [fifth lumbar vertebra]. Shiatsu students should go to old people's homes, you can learn many things about the origin of diseases there.'

'How was this?' He asks C, 'You had tension here?' He points to the lower back.

'You're right.' She says, 'I recognised the points where there was most tension, here and there.' She points, 'For me it is always difficult to sit so upright.' She demonstrates that she's sitting straight now: 'Afterwards it is much easier. I have the feeling that I have grown, I'm taller now and during the treatment I also had the feeling that I wanted to expand.'

'Still growing,' laughs Kishi, 'not yet finished. And you?' He points to the other person he had treated. 'Yes, I always had tension here and in the back.'

Another person asks, 'Maybe it doesn't happen to you, but to me it happens sometimes that people ask, *And what did you see?* at the end of a treatment.' Kishi thinks about it, then he replies:

'Never talk after a session and ask, *How was it?* It's very strange why you would ask this after feeling what took place. No *mon-shin*.[90] For me, after a session, if there's lots of talking, I feel that what I did was not a success. For me that would be the case, anyway. In Japan a certain kind of person asks many questions. First I give a session and then they ask, *And you, what did you see?* This is because the patient is attached to their pain; it's very important to them, *My pain, I'm very bad, I must show Kishi, please look at my pain.* If they have a funny feeling afterwards, a new feeling, then there is cure. But if they talk, always more comes. But I have no time for them to talk. The next patient will soon arrive; they have just 30 minutes. Maybe a different way is OK, I don't know.'

Someone comments from the class:

'Very often the reaction of the patient is that they have a very free head afterwards. In this situation I find it interesting not to talk afterwards but let them go out with this feeling. Maybe when they come for the next treatment and still want to talk about their reaction, then I'll talk about it.'

Kishi responds:

'I talk to patients about reactions myself. I give them a sheet of paper about possible reactions. How they might feel; feeling more or finding your real character. Or bad feelings or feeling tired. Some people's sensitivity does not wake up and that's very hard. I tell them

---

90 Mon-shin is talking diagnosis.

that maybe there will be elimination. For instance, the pee could be very dark, or the shit very smelly or there's a lot of it. My room smells bad after sessions because people are refreshed by their breathing changing. I have three fans in my practice room to get rid of the smell. People with cancer, in particular, have a peculiar smell. But it's very good for people to get it out. It's a good sign. Elimination shows on the skin sometimes, like an allergy, particularly if the liver is eliminating. But I tell them to leave it, it may last for three months, but please don't take drugs for it, no cortisone. Cortisone is bad for the kidneys. My work is the opposite of drugs; it cleans out. Don't stop this reaction.'

A student new to this work asks a question: 'So in this understanding, do you think that cancer is a symptom manifesting?' Kishi responds:

'Everyone has cancer. If you don't want life or you're not clear, or you are insensitive, if there's no elimination and no change, then cancer can grow. Seiki is not about curing cancer, but how to embrace life and to be alive even when you are "sick". To not be afraid. Death is natural, it's everywhere. Anyway, I decided in February 1980 on a simple life. Not big, not small, not born, not dead also. Nothing. The Buddha said this. Take off your armour. If you clarify yourself, your perception becomes clear and develops, if you do this, your natural character comes out. Maybe your true character is an artist, or writer or a business person or a spiritual person, anything. You are free. Nobody is making you do anything. I think this is the natural human. Many people think that to be natural is to be in a green space or on a mountainside, with clean air, eating vegetables. Perhaps live like a sheep. This is just an idea of health.'

A student agrees, 'I think it's most important to find what you really want. For me that is.' Kishi sits and is quiet for a while:

'Next year will be my workshop in Japan. It's very interesting. Some people come every time. They can't explain why they keep coming, they just want to. Or maybe it's stupid. But this is most important: not understanding. We need this. Gyoki is stupid. That's important. Shiatsu is stupid, but *in that moment* it's important. I think more of this is necessary. Please don't have fixed ideas about what Seiki is.'

SEI-KI: Life in Resonance – The Secret Art of Shiatsu

It is now nearing the end of the workshop and Kishi asks for questions. Someone says, 'You talk about being one with the other person, but for me, when I was doing Seiki, there were some areas where I felt I became one with my partner and then I would go to another place and suddenly there was no contact and in another place there was better resonance again.' He responds, 'No separation means one movement. Like two hands, like gyoki.'

Someone else says, 'I think I became more courageous on this workshop.' Kishi likes this: 'Yes, wilder. Seiki is wild, life philosophy.'

Another comments, 'The more I get the feeling of what you're talking about then it happens without me having to do very much and this is nice.' Kishi says, 'It's about quality. Seiki is quality contact.' There is a long pause and a quiet feeling in the room. Then Kishi asks the young boy, O, about his experience of Seiki with him. O says, 'First I didn't remember to breathe with you and it didn't work so well and then when I remembered to breathe with you, it went better.' Kishi listens carefully and O is very comfortable now in this room of adults, some of whom he has worked with. Kishi laughs, 'Now he *wants* to do it. On the first day and second day, this room had a different feeling. Now it's quiet. Noisy on the outside but...' He makes a sign, hands flat, 'the energy is more smooth.'

A new student wants to comment:

> 'This is the first time I met Kishi and for two days I was completely confused, I had all different feelings and I couldn't sleep at night. And today I have the feeling that what I'm taking with me from this workshop is that I don't have to become a Kishi clone or do it Kishi's way, I can take whatever I've learned in this workshop and integrate it into my work and see how the process goes. What I cannot take in, immediately, maybe I have to leave for now and see what will develop. It was a very beautiful experience and I'm sure it will go on.'

'Before, I gave Seiki to you,' Kishi says, in a gesture of offering, with his hands out, 'Now I take it back. This is my course. Please forget everything. Don't keep a fixed idea about it.' He pauses and sits quietly for a minute, 'But keep my influence behind you. Use *kyo* and move jitsu. Kyo is where? Here? Or here? It's like the wind. It's not necessary to understand it. Just feel.'

And one student asks, 'But what *is* kyo, what do you mean by *kyo?*' Kishi says, 'Using kyo.'

She asks again, 'But what is the *meaning* of kyo?' Kishi says, 'I don't know. I told you, it's not here, please.' Indicating a place on the body, 'Where is kyo? Kyo is in jitsu, jitsu is in kyo too. There is so much talking about kyo, kyo, kyo. It's not a discussion thing. Discussing it makes no sense. For me the point of Seiki is how to use kyo.'

Kyoko says, 'In Japanese this is gen*ki*. We say in Japanese, *o genki desu ka?* meaning *how are you?*, it refers to your original ki. But it's just a normal, everyday saying for us.'

A new student adds her thoughts:

'I want to say one more thing. I'm very moved. It's important to me to get real insight into the Japanese culture and understand Shiatsu, which I've been practising for 17 years. This morning I was very angry but now I am full of humility and gratitude. And I feel a big span between this endless depth and this human, very human being, this human doing, the way we are all trying to be in the world.'

An appreciative silence acknowledges her words.

Kyoko says:

'For me, because I'm married to Kishi, I have had the opportunity to come on many workshops. I see that people coming on workshops now feel something very quickly. It took me ten years to have this *sure* feeling. I'm glad that people come to it quickly. Some people said they don't feel the ki capsule that Kishi describes, but don't think like this. If you think like this, it becomes very hard and the joyful feeling of working together doesn't come so easily. Experience a nice feeling just in the moment; from moment to moment.'

People nod. Then she says, 'I understand what it's like to learn Seiki. I didn't train in Shiatsu, I'm not like Kishi. When I adjust people when they're doing gyoki, Kishi thinks my teaching is jitsu.' Everyone laughs. 'I think maybe if there is too much help, people don't like it. But I teach contact. I want to help because I understand that learning is a process and I understand this process because I had to go through it too.'

Another student says, 'I cannot imagine this workshop without Kyoko because there is a harmony with both together. It would be completely different without her.' Everyone readily agrees. Kishi laughs, 'Always Kyoko is talking, but me...' He is silent and smiles.

An old student of Kishi's says:

'I have to say that in this workshop I have felt very divided. It has touched me emotionally very much. On the one hand I'm a Shiatsu teacher and I want to understand something and I think it's wonderful that Kishi is writing a book. It's his development, but also good for Shiatsu. I have deep respect for this and I'm grateful. But it puts me into conflict with my teaching. And the other thing is about Seiki; I always enjoy this contact because I don't have to analyse it or put it into categories. But I recognise that this is the first time in 30 years of working with you that I really felt this so strongly and this is what I'm taking away with me. Thank you very much.'

Many Shiatsu therapists can sympathise with what the speaker has said. Another student nods and says quietly, 'I think that revolutions never pass by without pain. You must keep the way firmly in sight.'

The organiser himself now says:

'Thank you for coming. I was just saying before that many people have known Kishi for a long time. I first went on a workshop with Kishi in 1983 and it was very different from this. But your basic ideas were always the same, which is calling to your originality. On the outside there are many changes, but inside the essence is always... Kishi and Kyoko. So, thank you very much.'

Kishi is quiet for a while but puts his hand on his heart, 'Thank you for your nice words. I am touched.' At this point, many people are reaching for their handkerchiefs!

After noses are blown, Kishi says, 'Actually, this workshop might not have happened. After the first workshop, two weeks ago, the organiser said *please come here again*. We wondered about going somewhere else because this course was in doubt. But I'm glad we came here. Thank you very much.'

Everyone shares the bow and the workshop ends.

PART IV

MEETING KISHI

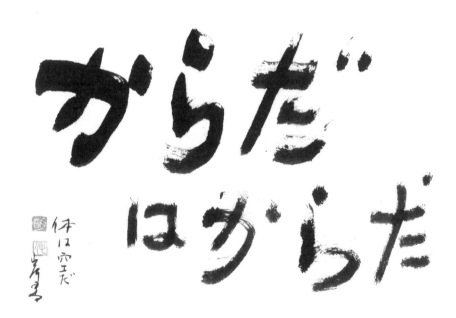

Karada wa Karada: the body is already empty
There is always the blue sky if you pass through the clouds.

(Calligraphy by Kishi)

Accounts of Seiki-Soho

Over the last few years, Kishi and Kyoko have collected accounts from people who have attended workshops and had private sessions, all over Europe. Others have been moved to write to Kishi of their own accord. What follows are a few of those accounts. Some are roughly translated or written by people for whom English is not their first language, but all give a flavour of how Seiki has touched people. They have found they can 'speak the body' very well.

My first experience with Kishi

When we started the class I felt OK, like always, that is, tension in my diaphragm but nothing more. Actually, I didn't know for sure if it was my diaphragm, I just had general tension just under my lung/heart zone. We started with gyoki. I was glad my hands were glowing warm like usual in this kind of exercise. When Kishi said that our lower bodies had to glow warm, I was really surprised. Mine didn't glow! I was worried because I normally have good sensibility in my body. I practised gyoki many times the same day, during the workshop and afterwards. The next morning I still didn't feel anything and I wanted Kishi to treat me, maybe this would solve something. So, when the moment arrived, I offered myself as a volunteer.

When Kishi first touched me I was nervous, I didn't know why. I simply was. Really quickly, my breathing relaxed when he put his hands on my shoulders. I lay face down. Kishi told the others that his hands were becoming very warm and mine were becoming cold. Suddenly my right hand felt a big stream of energy. My breathing became slower and the pressure in my back disappeared. Although the movement of Kishi's hands wasn't very spectacular, I suddenly felt my legs strong and warm. I felt a big change when Kishi touched me in my hara, my legs were becoming really warm and strong. It was very nice yet it was all physical, very nice but I wasn't changed in myself, my feeling self.

When I opened my eyes I noticed another change, I was there but my eyes were in a different place. I could not make contact with the rest of the people, like I was lower in my body. When I sat down I felt the change in my diaphragm, it was *loose*. My organs were moving down. It felt strange but a relief, actually it felt really nice. My body was rearranging itself. After fifteen minutes or so, I felt normal again but without tension and moving organs. Thank you very much for this experience, I won't forget this, at least my organs won't.

FVH, Belgium

Harmony and thankfulness

At the beginning of the treatment in seiza, I experienced Kishi's contact as firm and secure. After some oscillations, my breathing got better and he invited me to lie down. It's then when I got fascinated by the precision of his sense of finding my tensions and painful areas. Here I feel his contact with a great confidence and well-being. Although I do not feel katsugen, tensions get dissolved and they abandon me like the smoke Kishi talks about. He asks me to turn face up and his contact makes my breath wider, I feel liberation in my intention and I expand. My mind is amazed, observing Kishi's work, how he takes care of my needs, I feel he understands me, he releases knots, it's a process. He touches me here and there and he mentions something about my T-shirt that has the logo of Navarra's Shiatsu Association, he mentions something about my native city, Pamplona. Some touches later I disappear, I feel in limbo, I feel very fine and secure, I have no tensions, no hurry. Later, he brings me back to consciousness and, when I open my eyes, I feel something has happened, something very important but I wasn't there when it happened, I could be dead but

I feel very alive, pure, renovated, like I'm hollow inside. I experience harmony and thankfulness to Kishi for offering me that experience.

JM, Navarra

Scratching an itch

I felt that Kishi knew immediately where my body needed attention/ energy, and allowed it to happen like an itch you could not scratch; which you needed help from someone else to reach and allow to release. Thank you.

M, Banchory

An account of my treatment with Kishi sensei

I had a strange treatment with Kishi today during the class, I don't remember much about what he did except that he talked of the change of the seasons and of the weather, he also referred to sowing and reaping and laying fallow. I know the treatment lasted a long time but time passed quickly for me. Afterwards, I felt OK at first, and then it was time for a lunch break. I went into lunch but immediately felt that I should not eat; I tried drinking water but even that felt too much, so I went outside to find a place to be by myself for a while.

I went into the garden but could not settle. I stood on the bank outside the house and the wind seemed to come up the valley and blew straight through me. I felt this was very nice, so I thought maybe I need to walk in nature, and I started off across the field. Firstly I was walking then I was skipping and running, then I started to jump and shout out loud, by the end of the field I was jumping and shouting at the top of my voice!

I started to walk down the lane to the river and I felt so full of everything, I laughed and cried, I saw everything in the lane, the flowers and the weeds and it all looked so beautiful, so perfect and unique, everything was different and yet it all belonged together, a dragonfly flew past and then a butterfly, going before me down the lane.

On the wall opposite an old dog looked suspiciously at me. I went to the river and sat down to calm my mind and watch the water flowing, something bit me and I was roused from my reverie and decided to go back. On my way back up the lane the magic happened again. The flowers and the hedge looked so perfect, the dragonfly was still hovering, the sun shone and everything was radiant, as I passed by the dog I saw him wag his tail in greeting and I started to cry. I felt strangely accepted by this place. I felt like I belonged here and that there was no difference between myself, and the life around me and I was so grateful and so happy to be alive.

I remembered that Kishi had said, ' Looking with your eyes and your heart.'

Of course my body reacted to all this wonder and a few days later I passed several gallstones in the toilet, and felt as if life would have to change and never be the same again. I am very grateful to Kishi sensei for his inspirational teaching and help with healing my whole self.

With love and gratitude for the gift of life.

KC, Brighton

Connection with nature

After the treatment I felt silent, at peace and whole. Everybody was talking at tea break but I felt no words coming, my eyes and hands talk by themselves. There was too much noise for me but I needed friendly human contact, so I rested my head on G and found quietness; found the mother touch that I also felt during the treatment. I felt that the whole session was very feminine. I felt like a baby in her mother's arms, I felt softness and warmth, so much awareness. Felt the tensions as very precise knots, felt my mind sheered. I was observing from a deep place inside my belly, maybe from the uterus.

I felt the space inside and again my mind sheer and a connection with nature. I felt like a tree, like a lake surrounded by mountains, like an eagle, like a sea turtle. The pain in my lower back, which is quite old and deep, feels lighter, nearly gone and my knees a bit more happy. Thanks very much for your welcoming, for your precise, soft and firm touch.

SV, Segovia, Spain

Precision

Although Kishi had said that he worked without any pressure his treatment felt powerful and extremely precise.[91] In the beginning I was in my usual state of mind. But each time he said '...the breathing has changed...', I found myself going deeper into a dark yet comfortable space.

UH, Linden

Seiki: satisfied forever

The first Seiki treatment with Kishi caused a very warm feeling around my stomach. I felt nurtured, but not in a physical way. Wishes and desires muted. I felt complete, healthy and in my centre and I hope that feeling will stay forever.

UR, Nurnberg

Relaxed

We started in the sitting position. Kishi connected by holding my head just at the base of the neck. I suddenly felt a pain in my gallbladder, just for a few seconds. I then lay on my front and Kishi held a point on my head for a short while. He let go, then held again. My buttocks relaxed and my hips opened. At first I felt a little scared of letting go, then relaxed and felt safe with the comforting presence of Kishi. I lay on my back and Kishi held my neck, my hands twitched and I felt a coolness going through my body like rippling water. After the demonstration I had a headache for about 30 minutes, then felt much better and very happy. When I arrived home I observed that the whites of my eyes had become whiter.

AB

---

91 This is a partial misunderstanding: Kishi explains that pressure is not the point, contact is the point.

Waves

Kishi's presence (or resonance) held me awake while all boundaries became more blurred. I was 'in' my body yet my body had no physical sensation. Nothingness and breathing in and out like waves. Around my throat felt tingly and warm.

V

Cosy feeling

In the exercise with hands up, Kishi moved me and I had no centre and went easily sideways, backwards and forward. After he touched my lower back and I relaxed, I felt more centred more strength in my hara but, more and more with the treatment, I felt it as if my belly was filling more, very slowly. I felt air coming up to my mouth as it wanted to go out. I felt this many times. As Kishi was going through my body I felt my belly area getting slowly filled, very slowly as I was getting more relaxed. My attention was more and more in the belly as it was also getting warmer. From all parts of the body more to the centre. At the end, doing the same exercise with hands up I felt more strength in my hara, I could actually feel it because before this I had tried many times to take energy to the hara but always felt it not easy, especially on the right side. But now I could feel it and I also felt my breathing through my belly at the end. I sat with a feeling of the hara area warm and a very cosy feeling and my mind, my perception was clearer, I was breathing through this area, it was very warm.

Anon

Hello Kishi sensei and Kyoko san

I was the second person to be a volunteer body for Kishi to work on this evening. I have had back problems for 20 years and have had a back operation which has still left me with considerable pain. I fell over on the ice a couple of months ago and I have been having a lot of pain in my upper right arm, neck and jaw.

Kishi told me to sit with my back to him. The first place he touched was my upper right shoulder area and directly on the place where I had been having the most pain.

I felt warmth from Kishi's hands. He continued to gently hold my occipital area and a gentle swaying movement began, after a few seconds I felt like lying down and I lay on my stomach.

I let out a few deep exhalations as I was feeling a sense of release and movement of energy.

I heard Kishi tell the audience that I had shoulder tension; he went on to roll my head from side to side using his left hand on the base of my neck. I experienced this as a very welcome and opening sensation. My left leg rolled outwards and Kishi commented on this, showing the audience the movement my leg had made.

Kishi asked me to turn over onto my back. I had my eyes closed and I heard Kishi say that the ja-ki was leaving from my hara area quite forcefully. I felt a sense of relief and I opened and closed my mouth, really stretching my jaw which had been giving me pain all that day. I yawned I felt my arms move a little and also felt my legs jerking around.

Whenever my limbs moved it just felt right; I didn't really decide to make the movements, they happened spontaneously. At the end of the treatment, after bowing, I had the clearest feeling of a draft of air/energy exiting from the back of my head. I could feel the hairs standing on end and I giggled and put my hand over the area as I felt there may have been something stuck on my head. It was a very strong sensation of something coming out of my head.

Later, I shared my experience with the group and one lady put it to Kishi that it was necessary for him to be involved in order for me to have had my experience. Kishi responded by saying, 'What does he think of that?' So he was asking me to explain how I felt about the lady's comment.

My response was that from the initial touch to the feeling in my head at the end of the treatment, I had felt a great sense of gratitude, comfort, security and a sense of trust that I could just let myself go in the moment. A feeling of relief from tension and thinking, 'Yes, this is exactly where I want to be touched at this moment, thank you.'

Was that due to Kishi? Well yes, I suppose so, but the main thing I think is that I was there with pain and tension and a need for relief. Kishi 'heard' me and acknowledged me completely at that moment, for which I feel grateful.

TC

Seiki is in the interstices

It is in the gap between what we come up against and that which melts away on the touch.

It is cutting meat when the timing makes the flesh part on the slightest of touches. The knife does not come down hard. It does not push. It glides.

It is the heat between the hands in gyoki. The hands come together. Sweat forms in the fold. It expands and dissipates into the graininess of the atmosphere. This is environment. A canopy that holds together as one. A body connection that becomes a movement unfolding from a hidden point into a bearing.

It is automatic like a catapult. A spontaneous evolution like a leaf unfurling. This time of when to go and the going with it in a total commitment brings responsibility. It brings two-directional response. It leads to change. Because a certain phase in the way things are; a situation that one is in the ripple of the flesh, bunching up and slipping away again, has been noticed.

The eyes follow through from the alignment of the body that moves as one like a single snake vertebrae, from sacrum to occiput, through the pores of the skin opening out.

The smell, the breath, the small muscular groupings, the clenching of the anus, the hara, the throat, the valves of the heart, the lung, tendons in the knees, the calf muscle, the ankle and wrist tendons, the scapula jointing. All are orifices that open and close as a gauge to a wider association.

They work in conjunction with one another. They are echoes of one another. A voicing.

In that way we also course and filter though one another, through a reverberation of tendencies that work like a pump. The on-off of contact is this. It is gyoki or breathing between the hands. Building up the heat of proximity in the out-breath then allowing it to unfurl in the off touch – the in-breath.

The intervals. Seiki lives in these intervals creating a space of possibility. The space between cells.

To feel a constraint, go with it into its wringing turn like a spring tightening. To go with the disease or aggravation until at its extremity the rewind catches in.

This is automatic release when the body moves and the conscious human associations follow. This is thought-tendencies through and through with feeling response at every minute level of interest.

There is an intermingling and a conjoint intelligence which comes through. A deep compassion lasting.

There is a gathering and spreading simultaneously. A filtering system that nourishes every cell as each turns and jostles around another.

The body breaks and is remade. Not only once in a single trauma and cure but endlessly.

Life and death meet in the moment. In this gap is every different human possibility. A story is told.

RS, London

Sensitive to the breath

I felt that Mr Kishi was very sensitive to my breath. His hand is following my breath and giving it its space. But at the same time it is guiding my breath and giving it direction until, at some point, it's hard to tell who is leading; if my breath is moving his hand or his hand is moving me.

N, Israel

Seiki experience in Linden

When I decide to move to the futon for a Seiki demonstration, I suddenly feel my excited heartbeat. Inside of me it is vibrating. Before this all comes to my consciousness, Kishi's hand is already touching me between my shoulder blades. Again, I'm surprised and amazed how immediately he recognises my energy. I'm busy with my heartbeat and want it to calm down. I know it's the right timing for this Seiki demonstration. I feel my closedness, not ready for being touched and moved, even though Kishi's hand feels pleasantly warm and releasing. He asks me to lie down – again, right timing, I notice.

His hands are immediately there, touching my back. At the same time I have the feeling of touching myself! 'Ah, that's how it feels when I'm touching myself – I am in touch with me,' I think. Now I understand the image of the *empty mirror* which Kishi often uses. In Seiki I'm looking at myself (as in Shinto, I learn later that year in Japan). There is oneness, a non-differentiation. Together = to gather all that is separate.

When I lie on my back I feel tightness in the upper hara. Kishi confirms this. I so much desire to be soft. Then he touches my sternum. I feel that soon 'it will happen'. I want to give up, surrender to myself. My head moves – Kishi's hand touches my neck. I yield to his hand. Endless trusting and homecoming. His hand at the sternum is constant, deep and clear. Now the feeling changes. It becomes very quiet, internally and externally. Like the solar eclipse – a quieting or stillness of all movements for a moment that seems timeless. Before inhalation happens there is this feeling of stillness – this is transformation, I think afterwards. Feelings release. I start crying softly; then more intense. My body becomes an amoeba, tenses as one, holds the tension in one movement and then releases completely. I'm an amoeba in the ocean. It becomes peaceful, released, my heart relaxes and from its fullness it becomes empty.

Thank you, Kishi sensei, for this experience.

PS, Munich

Storm on an ocean

Kishi started to touch my sick parts (neck and shoulder blades where I have pain and no suppleness). Then there came a prickling in my face and navel. It went to my arms and it got worse and worse. That prickling went down to my hara. It felt in my hara as a storm on an ocean. I had the feeling that my hara went up and down, from the left to the right. That feeling was very strong. My whole body was full of energy. I've never had such an experience. Kishi said that the woman in me was not developed. I know that it was true, just as all the other things he said.

MS

New life

I feel like a new life starts now, huge amounts of old 'rubbish' (Kishi's word) seemed to be leaving my body. *Old* stuck energy from who knows where, being pulled from the top of my head by Kishi's hand, from my chest, from my abdomen. I am now feeling a huge sense of calm, relief and opening as I sit drinking a cup of three year tea, while chatting with Kishi and D and writing down my impressions. Thank you.

JM

Dear Kishi, Dear Kyoko

Only when I was home I realised how strong was the influence of this few days with you working with us. All of a sudden I felt my heart being full of LOVE. In this moment I saw and felt YOUR LOVE and I was deeply moved. In my body I felt the change of my breathing. It was slow, deep, full and down into the hara. My legs felt light, my hara full and strong. I know I cannot keep this state but I tasted something beautiful I can work for. Thank you for all you gave to us.

CB

Part of me

I thank you for your kindness, your calm and for your healing heart. You have facilitated me to remember how important it is to carry out our inner heart when treating someone. But I should not have said, 'treated', I prefer to say what I felt yesterday during the session at school that it, 'to breathe with someone, to have a speech between hearts.' At first, during the past few days, I supposed that Seiki was something apart from me. Instead I found out that Seiki could be part of me.

AF, Rome

My experience of Seiki

I wanted to improve the stiffness and the pain of the muscles of my left shoulder and my head so I went for a Seiki session.

Since I did not think that there could be a strong curative effect with weak pressure, I was very surprised by the effect and skill, the emotional strength and the concentration. As for the Shiatsu and the manual therapeutics that I received up to now, it was common to receive pressure (on muscles and body surface) to some extent, and receive superfluous support occasionally. It thought that this was suitable as a method for removing pain and cori (stiffness).

However, Seiki was surprising in that it is a practical technique which treats with a sense of breathing completely, without totally applying stress to the body.

I did not feel this as a point but there was a sense of stroking which touched me and the pressure was transmitted as a field.

It was comfortable pressure which was united with the partner's breathing and warmth slowly comes.

It pulls out the balance and pliability of the body and makes muscles relax in addition to the operation which moves a joints slowly.

And at the same time, spiritual relaxation was also felt and I actually felt that it was the wonderful skill in which mind and body could make a pain improve. Although it seems easy enough to describe Seiki in words, I thought that remarkable experience and moral self-discipline were required as practice to learn the skill that leads to these effects so far.

YU, Japan

A Seiki session

So this is where I propose to start – with a Seiki session. Look through my eyes.

Like a kind of dance, an invitation is offered by Kishi to work with him, whether for free or paid, and this is met by a desire to participate from some person.

The pair will usually kneel on a futon and bow to each other Japanese style starting off the connection with mutual acknowledgement and respect.

First, contact isn't rushed, time is given to see the person, their body, breathing, small movements, holding patterns. No need to rush. Then the first touch, often but not exclusively, on the top of the shoulders near the base of the neck. There are no rules but this place offers good opportunities to enter into connection.

A few moments breathing together, intense observation given to subtle changes. Seeing.

Perhaps some guided gentle movement of the head around the neck, or of the whole upper body and the person relaxes down, appearing to enter into an almost trance-like state.

The position may change now, either naturally by the person, or on Kishi's request, usually to lie on their front, and work will proceed on the back.

Where to start? Again no rush, no busy-ness, no doing.

Kishi's hand or hands will move to their next place of contact, perhaps for just a few seconds touch, perhaps longer. Enough to achieve their work.

The various areas of the spine and sacrum may be of most interest, but again there is no form, no pattern for the head to follow, anywhere might be the most important point for the next moment. The hands know.

And contact might be maintained without touch, off the body simply using ki from the hands or even from the eyes.

Then on to the person's front, the abdominal region, the hara in Japanese culture usually taking the most attention, along with the occiput at the base of the skull. But still any place where the body is holding may be the next place – the solar plexus, the base of the sternum, the heart area, below the throat.

And the body will respond.

There may be subtle spontaneous movements, or even less than subtle ones as the body enters into what has been called katsugen in Japanese culture. A state in which the natural ability and intelligence of the body to release stress and balance by itself becomes active.

External expression might be dramatic at times, physical shaking, laughter or the primal scream, but is not given attention or judged; value instead being placed on the internal ki process that is going on within the body as it moves towards a more harmonious state of being.

Space is given when the person needs it.

Kishi once described such a moment as like a mother looking after a baby: protecting, giving full attention, taking total care, but at the same time allowing and giving freedom without judgement. Acceptance.

A sudden change in the breathing, often the deep inhale, what I would call 'the breath of life', when a single full unrestricted breath is suddenly taken, signals the end of a previous state of being and entry into something new.

Ja-ki coming out, the release of stagnant energy, may be indicated by Kishi from some point of the body, with his visual description of it, as a kind of dark smoke. Some see it, some don't.

And so the session comes to a close indicated not by the clock, but by the completion of the process. The body having changed to the extent it can at that time. A natural end.

Both people will usually bow to each other again and then part and few words will be spoken.

But from my own experience as a recipient, there is a feeling of warmth and connection in the contact which is enough.

So this is all I see – how do we go beyond this to communicate what this work really is?

FA, Brighton

POSTSCRIPT

I did not write this book in order to criticise anyone. It has been 40 years since I first learned Shiatsu and 30 years since I started to call my work *Seiki*. For 10 years before starting Seiki I had met and learned with much respect from the two great masters of Shiatsu, Namikoshi and Masunaga. Both were very active during this time and it was the golden age of Shiatsu in Japan. It was a wonderful time for me to be a student of Shiatsu and it was also time for Shiatsu to leave its nest in Japan and spread to different parts of the world. I also left my nest, and I left Shiatsu.

Master Masunaga especially had a big influence on me. But in order to listen to my inner voice and find my own path, it was necessary to leave everything I had learned. I searched and explored this 'wild life philosophy'. I called it Seiki and continued the search which led to Seiki-Soho. Europe became the base for my work.

There have been people who sympathised and connected with Seiki and also those who have left. In the meantime, Shiatsu has spread to many parts of the world and has changed. Now Shiatsu has become clearer to me from the Seiki perspective. With the conviction of Seiki-Soho I feel that the time has come to compile my life's work.

I can say that Seiki was born in Japan and nurtured in Europe. That is why this book is written through Alice Whieldon from the United Kingdom.

I would like to thank the people, especially in Europe, whom I have met in person, and also whom I have met indirectly through contacts, and dedicate this book to them.

Akinobu Kishi
Maebashi, Japan
January 2011

GLOSSARY

Please note that the words listed are given only approximate and fairly literal translations for the purpose of immediate reference. In using the glossary bear in mind that the context-specific meanings of these words are much broader and richer than it is possible to convey here.

Anma and Koho Anma   Anma is the traditional manual therapy of Japanese using meridians and Anpuku. Due to restrictions in the use of Anpuku during the Edo era, it introduced complicated techniques and its facility for curing illness diminished. The early form was called Koho Anma and its method of hosya is different from Masunaga's Shiatsu.

Anma-Doin   When the Chinese brought Doin-Ankyo to Japan, the Japanese developed it in their own way and this is what it became known as.

Anpuku   Manual hara treatment.

bo-shin, mon-shin, bun-shin, setsu-shin (sesshin)   The four diagnostic skills of Kanpo. Sesshin is the essence of Masunaga's Shiatsu and leads to 'life-sympathy'.

chakusyu   The place where the practitioner's hands first land.

Doin-Ankyo   An early form of manual therapy that the Chinese introduced to Japan.

Fuku-Shin   Diagnosis through touch, similar to Anpuku, advocated by Todo Yoshimasu.

gassyo-gyoki 'Breathing by hand' with the hands in the prayer position – one of the possible exercises for developing sensitivity and preparing the hands for wa-ki in Seiki.

gyoki-hachiriki Gyoki with movements derived from the Waraku martial art.

hara Anatomically the abdomen, central to Japanese culture and spirit.

hibiki Echo/life-sympathy (between the hands in two-handed Shiatsu).

hosya *Ho* touch is for kyo and *sya* touch is for Jitsu; ho compensates a deficient point but, in fact, like yin/yang, ho/sya cannot be separated and form an ever-moving relationship.

Iokai Shizuto Masunaga's Shiatsu institute.

ja-ki A phenomenon which arises in the process of kyo/jitsu balancing; the dregs left by movement and a sign of change.

Judo Kappo Judo Seifuku or Bonesetting – a form of physiotherapy.

Kanji The traditional Chinese characters used in the Japanese writing system.

Kanpo (Eastern medicine) Kanpo is the traditional Japanese medicine which developed in Japan, in a unique form, from the medicine of ancient China. It was formalised during the Edo period (1600–1867). Kanpo is different from Chinese medicine which continued to develop in its homeland. In Japan it is called 'Eastern medicine' as opposed to 'Western medicine'. Today 'Kanpo' often refers only to herbal medicine.

katsugen Regenerating movement; katsugen, so named, comes from Noguchi's Seitai and was derived from Shinto practices of a shamanic nature that came out of norito recitation.

keiraku Meridian.

ki Ki leads to resonance of a life.

ki-do-ma Ki is timing, do is quantity, ma is space. It is a term used in various fields and the three elements are different; ki-do-ma in Seiki is right timing, right place and when to finish.

Koho Classical.

kokoro Heart.

kotodama The Japanese idea that words or sounds have a particular spiritual power.

kyo/jitsu A phenomenon resulting from distortion of mind/body in a living body.

ma-ai The suitable distance and timing between people.

Moxibustion The application of heat to points on the body, directly or indirectly through burning the herb, mugwort.

mu-shin Selflessness.

norito Shinto recitation.

Seitai This has a number of different forms in Japan but is, broadly, a system of exercises and therapy.

seiza The traditional way of sitting in Japan, on the knees.

sekkei An element of Acupuncture sesshin.

setsumyaku Acupuncture pulse diagnosis and part of Acupuncture sesshin.

Shinto The native, folk religion of Japan.

Suiatsu Fusai Ota's manual therapy; the skill of Anpuku.

syo (sho) diagnosis (syoshindan) Classical Eastern diagnosis; that part of cure which understands what a patient's life wants and acts, simultaneously, as therapy. It is not diagnosis through naming a disease.

tanden Lower abdomen but, like hara, this has a much broader meaning.

tekiatsu   Appropriate touch in Shiatsu.

tsubo   Usually translated as 'point'; often Acupuncture points.

wa-ki   Gyoki breathing by hand, performed with a partner in Seiki sessions.

Waraku   A martial art in the tradition of Kotodama-Turugi in the Shinto sect, Oomoto, Japan, developed by former Karate champion, Maeda sensei.

Zen   Concentration of spirit going into the state of selflessness, or the abbreviation for the Zen sect in Buddhism.

APPENDIX I

FLOWCHART OF THE HISTORY OF TRADITIONAL JAPANESE FOLK MEDICINE

Key

------- indirect links

———— direct links

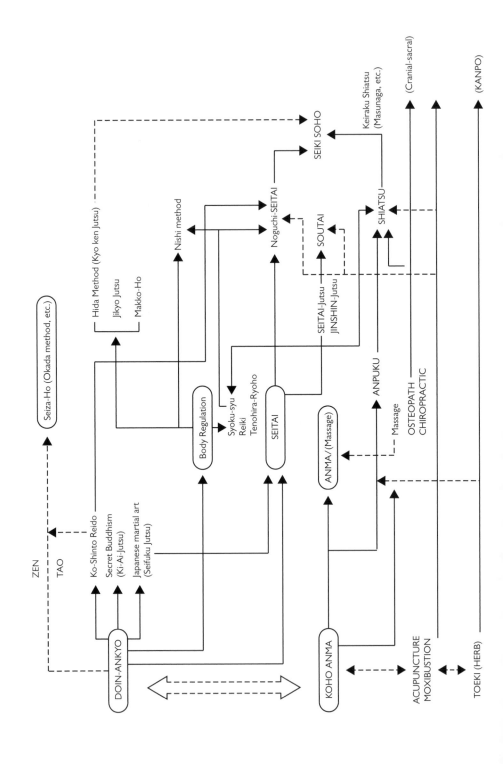

APPENDIX II

DR TARO TAKEMI'S ARTICLE ON THE NEED FOR KANPO

This article by Dr Taro Takemi, from Eastern Medicine (edited by Takao Otsuka, 1973), was translated and summarised by Kyoko Kishi. Taro Takemi was highly influential in the revival of Kanpo since he was the chief medical authority in Japan and advocated taking Kanpo seriously such that, today, medical students can usually study modules in Eastern medicine alongside their scientific studies. It was because of his research and recommendations that the Institute of Oriental Medical Research at Kitazato University was established where Masunaga sensei later became a professor.

Nowadays doctors study medicine in the German style and structure, so Western medicine underlies all medicine in Japan. Already, Kanpo is considered to be little more than a fairy story in medicine. However, I did lots of research and in my clinical practice I met with various problems that this medical approach could not address. But, when they were addressed with Kanpo, I can confirm that the cures effected were sometimes miraculous. One of my patients was the famous novelist, Kōda Rohan (1867–1947), who introduced me to several books on Kanpo and instructed me in the essence of Kanpo medicine. At that time I was still studying the medical application of physics in the Institute of Physical and Chemical Research and this came like a bolt from the blue. Speaking to Mr Rohan, he was very critical about medicine and I listened carefully to him and realised that he was saying things to which I must pay attention. He spoke about the basic premise that, while we are alive, all the complicated operations of protecting ourselves have an effect on the body. Kanpo medicine looks at how this manifests in the patient and is a medicine of intuition. We already have many ways to cure ourselves inside and Kanpo is how to bring this mechanism out and encourage our own healing, while modern medicine just attacks the symptoms.

This medicine by the intuition which Mr Rohan talked about, haunted me and affected me very deeply. Listening to my friend's experience and those of his acquaintances and the discussion of various other cases, I understood that, in Kanpo medicine, diagnosis and therapy are one. In contrast with analytic Western medicine, Kanpo medicine (herbal medicine) is synthesised by intuition and considers medication according to this synthesis gathered and understood by the doctor. It is inherently different in every case. Kanpo is not based on diagnosis through blood analysis and X-ray, etc.; the doctor uses the five senses and considers a patient's illness subjectively by understanding their mind rather than through test results. I could appreciate this.

It is also clear that in Kanpo, individual differences in the mechanism of the onset of disease is considered. It seems that the basis of Kanpo medicine is treatment rather than research. Cure is important but, in Western medicine, there is not so much interest in the person as in the condition. In Kanpo, integrated intuitive observation is the starting point in curative medicine. Even if oral consultation, ocular inspection, palpation, etc. in Western medicine are the work of the same five senses, they are not used to directly relate to what is being analysed – the patient – while a feature of Kanpo medicine is that it is directly interested in the patient.

Moreover, it differs from Western medicine in the value given to the effect of observation valuation. Kanpo medicine views the attitude of human understanding as its base, which originally came from Chinese philosophy.

Also in Western medicine, the wonderful achievements of psychological research, like that of Jung, have more recently emerged so we see that Western medical science investigates every aspect of the human being to the last. In this respect I think that Western psychology and Eastern thinking come close together.

Although I do not know Kanpo well myself, I do believe that this approach is important and must not be neglected. Also, when I went to the research institutes of drug companies in Germany and Switzerland, it turned out that they are researching Eastern medicine very seriously and I came across four or five foreigners who could read Eastern medical books while I was there.

I keenly realised the immediate importance of establishing a Foundation for Oriental Medicine Research and was very happy that the head of the Kitazato Institute accepted my idea and I was thus able to influence the establishment of the Foundation for Eastern Medicine Research as part of the Kitazato Institute. The aim there will not be that of looking for a particular medicine for a particular illness, as is done in Europe, but of researching Kanpo as a whole in its unique form. I would hope we would make some interesting new discoveries. We must not expect instant results though. I think that Kanpo and Western medicine can be naturally integrated at such a research institute where our common purpose is a new life science expressly for the purpose of the survival of humanity.

ACKNOWLEDGEMENTS

Kyoko Kishi's dedication and patience has been crucial to this book. It could not have been written without her. My parents and step-parents have been unstintingly supportive too. My writing group in Ontario, Canada, enveloped me with lovely warmth and encouragement. Paul Lundberg, Mark Burton and Frankie Jaggs are kind Seiki friends who listened to me for many hours, read early drafts and helped keep me sane. My Seiki friends in Europe have given me places to stay, kept me fed and boosted my morale over various trips to meet with Kishi and Kyoko. I thank them all from the bottom of my heart. Our publisher, Jessica Kingsley, was a great find and said just the right things at just the right times. I could not have hoped for better.

Alice Whieldon

INDEX

Page numbers in *italics* refer
to illustrations

Acupressure 66
Acupuncture 14, 30, 32
    n32, 45, 79
    Association 42
    charts 66
    China 11
    Daikoku 25
    diagnosis 40
    theory 41
    sesshin 42, 45
    Shiatsu 66
    Masunaga 61, 63–4, 66,
        131
    meridians 66
Agricultural University,
    Tokyo 47
Aikido 120 n79, 133 n88,
    134
anatomy 17–19, 22, 34, 72
Andrews, Clifford
    Quantum Shiatsu 5 n3
Anma 17, 20, 22–3, 25–7,
    29–30, 42, 65, 73,
    82, 131
    Anma-Doin 12, 63
    Fusai Ota 22
    Koho Anma 12, 14–17,
        20, 22, 32, 40, 44,
        64–5, 72, 131–2
    Masunaga 40, 60, 106
    Namikoshi 33
    rikan no jutsu 126
Anma-Doin *see* Anma
Anpuku 15–17, 20, 22–3,
    25–6

Anpuku-Doin *13*, 126
Anpuku-Zukai 13, 22, 26
    Chinese 66
    Masunaga 40
    Namikoshi 33
    Fusai Ota 106
    Japanese medicine 132
    Kishi 128
    Koho Anma 131
    Shiatsu 82, 131
appaku-ho 73
    see also pressure/pressing
armour 94–5, 106, 108,
    141
Art of War, The 116, *117*
atsu-hansya 72
attachment 73, 90, *91*, 101–
    3, 107, 110, 116

bi-chi 96
Bonesetting 46
bo-shin 78
bow 107, 121–2, 126–7,
    129, 133–4, 138, 144,
    152, 158–9
breath/breathing *89*, 90 n69,
    92, 97–8, 101–5, 107,
    109–10, 112–13, 115,
    118, 121, 125–30, 133,
    135–8, 141–2, 146–7,
    150–1, 153–4, 156–9
    breathing again 8, 88–118
Buddhism
    Buddha 141
    Medicine 60
    Monks 10, 52 n49
    Religion 15
    Sutra 60 n53

bun-shin 78

calligraphy *58, 89, 91, 95,
    96, 98, 99, 100, 117,
    119, 145*
cats 97
chakusyu 107
China 10–12, 14
Christianity 17
*Chronicles of Japan (Nihon
    Shoki)* 10
Chuang-Tzu 114, 118
concentration, mental
    Kishi 173, 84, 98, 109,
        122, 125, 132–5,
        157
    Masunaga 70, 73–5, 78,
        125
    Namikoshi 72, 74
    Shiatsu 73, 135–6
Confucius 15
cure 94, 106, 131, 168

Daigyou, Yoshio Dr 28–9,
    31
Daikoku, Sadakatsu 25, 71
Dejima 18
desire 93–5, 105, 107,
    108–9, 112–3, 132
diagnosis 11, 16, 40, 69,
    72, 76, 79
    Acupuncture 40
    back 65, 80
    Eastern 60, 78
    hara 80
    kyo/jitsu 65, 68, 72
    Masunaga 86
    medical 76

syo diagnosis 45, 64–5,
    67, 70, 74, 77–9,
    84, 87, 92, 98, 131
syoshindan 79, 106
    see also hara
discipline 7, 65 n56, 80–1,
    84, 157
distortion 77, 90, 92–3, 95,
    98, 111–12, 134
Do 46
    see also Way
Doin-Ankyo 12

echo see hibiki
Edo 14, 15, 16, 18, 22
ego 97
Endo, Ryokyu 14 n13
enlightenment (satori) 71
    n60, 108–9
eshin 55
    see also enlightenment;
    satori

focus see concentration,
    mental
Freud 65
Fujii, Dr 27, 86
fuku-shin 20, 21
    see also hara, diagnosis
furube see katsugen

Galen 18
God 7 n4, 77, 127–8,
gyoki 90, 101, 107, 109,
    124, 126, 133, 138–9,
    141, 142–3, 146, 153,
    154
gassyo 109, 127–8, 134,
    137
hachiriki 133–4

hachiriki see gyoki
hakama 120
hara 15, 16, 93 n72, 109,
    130, 136–7, 147,
    151–3, 155–6, 158
    diagnosis 20, 22, 80
    treatment 15, 22, 128,
    130–2

Haratori 15, 20
healing 94
health 10–11, 20, 22, 25,
    34, 50, 52, 70, 93–5,
    105–6, 110–11, 113,
    125, 127, 141
heart see kokoro
Heian period 15
herbs, medical 12, 14
    see also Kanpo
hibiki 68, 81, 134
Hirata, Kurakichi 24 n21,
    38 n38–9, 122
    zone 122
ho-ho 40
hosha see hosya
hosya 77, 80, 93
humours 18

Ikematsu, Shigeyuki 25
instinct 53, 107
intuition 67, 78, 82–3, 107,
    168
Iokai 37, 42–3, 45, 48, 52,
    54, 60, 64, 67, 70–1,
    73, 82, 87, 135
ishin-ho 12
Izawa, Tadashi 25

ja-ki 92, 115–6, 122, 125,
    128–30, 138–9, 152,
    159
Japan
    arts 7, 10, 49
    culture 11, 12, 15, 92, 95
    isolation 12, 18
    medieval 12
Japan Shiatsu College 30,
    33–4, 36, 41, 47, 59,
    60, 65–5, 71–2, 111
    see also Namikoshi,
    Tokujiro
jiriki 84
jitsu 68, 70–1, 73, 76, 78,
    80, 84, 92, 111, 134,
    138, 142–3
Judo 46
Judo Kappo 30, 46, 132
Jung, Carl 168

jyo-kyo ka-jitsu 93

Kagawa, Genetsu 20
kami 7
kanji 5 n2, 75, 125
Kanpo 19, 20, 34, 45, 60,
    63, 65, 67, 167–9
karada 145
Karate 46, 133 n88
Kato, Fusajiro 30
katsugen 53–4, 92, 109,
    110–11, 115–6, 127,
    129, 132, 147, 159
katsugen undo 53
kengyou 16–17
keriaku see meridian
ki 66, 90, 92, 94, 97, 107,
    112–13, 115, 134
    capsule 92, 122, 130,
    132, 134
    culture 81, 87, 104, 116,
    132
    original 143
    passing 90, 98, 102, 104,
    112, 118
    regulating 5 n2
    Seiki 84
    use 19
    see also resonance
ki-do-ma 112
Kiriyama, Kinzo 30
Kishi, Akinobu
    co-author 5–6
    biography 46–55
    Japan Shiatsu College 48
    katsugen 53–4
Masunaga 29, 45, 48–52,
    54–5, 57, 59–87
Namikoshi 47–8, 57
Paris 49–51, 82
Seiki 5 n2, 6
Shiatsu 7, 26, 55
Kitazato University 44, 167,
    169
koan 38
kokoro 71, 79, 98, 99, 101,
    108, 114
Korea 11
koshi 135

kotodama 71, 101, 133 n88
Koyama, Zentaro 25, 36
Kuriyama, K. 24 n21
kyo 68–70, 73, 76, 78, 84,
   111, 134, 138, 142–3
kyo/jitsu 69, 73, 81, 111
   balance 68, 76–7, 92
   character 68
   distortion 77
   following 79
   hosya 65, 80, 93
   life-sympathy 68
   looking for 68
   Masunaga 65, 67, 73,
      84, 111
   meridians 67-8
   Namikoshi 72
   Seiki 69, 76, 90, 111,
      128
   sesshin 68
   see also diagnosis, kyo/
      jitsu

life-sympathy 67–8, 70, 75,
   77–8, 80–1, 84–5,
   97, 134

ma 95
ma-ai 98, 102
Maeda 133 n87
magic 18, 106
manual therapy 10–12,
   14–16, 20, 22, 25–6,
   29, 31–2, 43, 61, 84,
   86, 131
   Hirata 39, 122
   Kishi 46, 55, 124
   Masunaga 36, 40, 60,
      63–5, 82
   Namikoshi 33
martial arts 46, 109, 120,
   133
   hara 16
massage 20, 23, 46
Masunaga, Shizuka 36
Masunaga, Shizuto 26, 29,
   30, 31–2, 34, 86
   biography 36–45

Kishi 29, 45, 48–52,
   54–5, 160
Namikoshi 37, 40
Noguchi 54
revolution 81–2, 87
Sasaki 5 n3
teaching 37–3, 61
The Shiatsu Treatment 86
Matsumoto, Betto 99
medicine
   Chinese 11, 12, 19, 22,
      41–2, 63, 65–7, 72,
      91, 131
   conventional 106
   Eastern 10, 65, 71–2, 82,
      167, 169
   Education 12, 14, 18
   folk 10, 12, 66
   Japanese 32, 41–2, 61,
      65–6, 68, 79
   politics 16
   revolution 37, 81–2,
      87, 93
   Seiki 95
   soul 65, 82
   traditional 64
   traditional Chinese
      medicine (TCM) 11
      n7, 41
   Western 17–20, 26, 76,
      78, 169
meditation 53, 75
Meiji 20
   Emperor 100
meridian 64, 66, 69, 72,
   79, 81, 84–5, 104,
   131, 134–5
   Japan Shiatsu College 72
   kyo/jitsu 67
   map/chart 42, 67–9,
      71–2, 85, 128
   Masunaga 40, 42, 60,
      65–71, 77, 81,
      84–6, 93
   philosophy 42, 65, 70,
      81, 86
   recognition/seeing 66,
      79, 81

misogi 53
mon-shin 78, 140
Moxibustion 11, 14, 30, 32
   n32, 45, 66, 131
mu-shin 68, 75–6, 81, 85,
   92, 96, 102, 107

Naikan 65
Namikoshi, Tokujiro 24
   n21, 26, 29, 30, 32,
   69, 71–3, 74, 81, 86,
   111
   biography 33–5
   Kishi 47–8, 50, 55, 57,
      160
   Masunaga 36–7, 40, 69,
      71
   teaching 40, 43, 61
   see also Japan Shiatsu
      College
Nara period 11
Nihon Shoki (Chronicles of
   Japan) 10
Noguchi, Haruchika 53–4,
   131–2
noh theatre 95
no-mind see mu-shin
norito 53 n51, 133

obstetrics 20, 22
occiput 121–3, 153, 158
Ogawa, T 32 n32
Ohashi, Wataru 44, 60 n53
   Sasaki 5 n3
   see also Zen Shiatsu
Oomoto 133 n88
Oriental Medical Research,
   Institute of 44, 167,
   169
Ota, Fusai 13, 22, 25, 26,
   106

pain 33, 39 n37, 47, 69,
   80–1, 102, 105, 110,
   125, 139–40
parasympathetic nervous
   system 29
pathology 65, 68

philosophy
  alternative 50
  Chinese 12
  differences 19
  Eastern 17, 31–2, 37, 39,
    63, 65, 111
  Japanese 10, 41, 76, 131
  Masunaga 111
  meridian 65, 70
  health 22, 28, 34
  Western 37, 63
  wild 95, 142, 160
physiology 17, 34, 72
physiotherapy 46
points 11 n8–9, 25, 33–4,
  40, 66–7, 69, 72, 79,
  107, 112–13, 115,
  118, 125–6, 130, 150
  see also tsubo
pressure/pressing
  finger 23
  Kishi 74, 132, 150, 157
  Masunaga 40, 64, 68,
    73–4, 81, 84, 135
  Namikoshi 33–5, 72, 74
  Namikoshi and Masunaga
    40, 71, 74
  perpendicular 73, 79,
    125, 136
  Shiatsu 92, 102, 115,
    157
  stationary 22
printing press 15
psychology 36–7, 41, 59,
  65, 82, 169
psychotherapy 41, 65

Red Book, The 24
reido see katsugen
religion 18
resonance 83–4, 90, 92–3,
  97, 101, 104, 106–8,
  110, 112, 115, 118,
  138
  see also ki
rikan no jyutsu see Anpuku,
  Anpuku-Doin
Rikyu 84
Rogers, Carl 41, 65

Rohan, Koda 167–8

sacrum 108, 128, 139, 153
Sasaki, Pauline 5 n3
  Ohashi 44
  Shiatsu 5
Sato, Koji 75
satori (enlightenment) 71,
  108
  see also eshin
science 10, 18, 22, 26–7,
  29, 63, 67, 72, 76, 78,
  82, 169
Seiki 6
  aim 94
  kanji 5 n2
  Kishi 69, 83
  Shiatsu 5, 86
  soho 7, 55, 57, 87–8, 90,
    97, 92, 97, 111–12,
    114–16, 125, 129,
    132, 160
  workshop 5, 55, 61, 88,
    98, 104, 111, 115,
    118, 119–144, 146
Seitai 24 n21, 25, 53–4,
  131–2
  Jutsu 132
  Soho 12 n12
seiza 65, 120–1, 126, 130
sekkei 63–4, 67, 84, 134
Sekkotsu see Judo Kappo
selflessness see mu-shin
serenity 90, 97, 101–102,
  107, 109, 117 n78
sesshin 58, 67, 73–4, 76,
  78–81, 84
  acupuncture 63
  diagnosis 67
  Kishi 97
  Masunaga 40–2, 45, 60,
    64, 67–71, 75, 77–
    81, 83–4, 92, 97,
    128, 131, 134–5
  setsu-shin 128
  Zen 75
  see also diagnosis
setsumyaku 63
setsu-shin see sesshin

Shiatsu
  aims 94
  Anma 17
  College, London 6
  conversations about
    59–87
  diagnosis 22
  fusion 79
  hara 16, 22
  history 7, 9–46
  Japanese 128, 131
  Japanese arts 7
  Kishi 6–7, 92
  license 27–30
  Masunaga 92, 135
  meridian 67, 77, 85
  principles 30, 48, 51, 60,
    69, 73–4, 76, 83,
    85–6, 124, 135–6
  Quantum 5 n3
  Seiki 5
  Tao, 14 n13
  Western/European 45,
    66, 69, 73, 81–2,
    128, 131
Shiatsu Institute of Therapy
  33
Shiatsu Institute, Tokyo 33
Shiatsu-Ho 23
Shinran 52
shinsen-jitsu 77
shin-shin ichi-nyo; mind/
  body is one 62
Shinto 7, 14–15, 31, 51–3,
  53 n51, 133, 155
sho see diagnosis, syo
shoshindan see diagnosis,
  syoshindan
shoulder 103, 109, 121–2,
  146, 152, 157–8
  blades 107, 134, 155
Society of Eastern Medicine
  82
soho 102
  Seitai 12 n12
  see also Seiki
solar plexus 93, 123, 137
Sotai 132

soul 110
  see also medicine
spirituality 20, 108–9, 111,
  116, 127, 141, 157
stagnation 8, 95, 106, 112,
  116, 159
stimulation 73, 112, 125
  Acupuncture 93
  Anma 22, 73
  Anpuku 22
  Hirata 39 n37
  Seiki 94, 98
  Shiatsu 81
suffering 31, 107
Sugiyama, Major General 36
Suiatsu 22, 106
Sun Tzu 116, *117*
surrender 53, 84, 155
sya-ho 40, 71, 80
sympathetic nervous system
  29
symptoms 29, 78, 106–7,
  168
syo diagnosis *see* diagnosis,
  syo
syoshindan *see* diagnosis,
  syoshindan

Takagi, R. 24 n21
Takemi, Taro Dr 44 n41
tanden 93
Taoism 31, 114
tariki 84, 112
Tea Ceremony 7, 84–5, 95
Teate 20, 68
tekiatsu 68, 74, 77, 80–1
Tenpeki, Tamai 23, *24*,
  25–6, 29, 33, 36, 71
Three Minute Shiatsu 34
Toho-Binran *21*
Tokugawa Shogunate 14
transmission 14, 26, 43, 60
treatment 11, 63, 69, 72,
  79, 104–5
tsubo 63, 66, 72, 73, 81
Tsukuda, Takichi 24
Tuina 66

Ueshiba 133 n88
unconscious 92, 107, 110,
  112, 133, 139

wa-ki 90, 94, 107, 109,
  132, 139
Waraku 133
Way (*Do*) 46 n46, 55, 85,
  114

Yamaguchi, Hisayoshi 31
Yasuyori, Tamba 12
yawn 103, 110, 127–8,
  134, 137–8, 152
yin/yang 71
yoga 12, n12
Yoshimasu, Todo 20, *21*

zazen 75
Zen 31, 38, 49, 65, 75, 80
Zen Shiatsu 44, 60 n53, 71,
  75–6
zui-syo 79